Life Giving Dementia Care

Let's Talk: How to Bring Confidence,
Compassion and Joy into Your Role as a Caregiver

Toni Kanzler

ISBN: 978-1-7361797-0-3 (paperback)
ISBN: 978-1-7361797-1-0 (ebook)
Library of Congress Control Number: 2020923749

Cover design by Angie Ayala, pro_ebookcovers
Editing by Sky Nuttall
Formatting by Polgarus Studio

DOWNLOAD YOUR FREE CAREGIVER CHECKLISTS NOW!

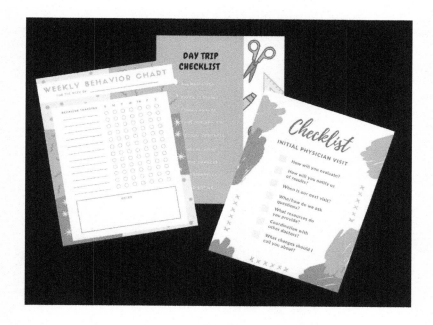

PLEASE READ THIS FIRST

I quickly learned that checklists were my best friend as a caregiver.

To say a GIANT thank you for investing in my book, I'd love to offer you instant access to three caregiver checklists.

They will help you successfully begin your journey in

LIFE GIVING DEMENTIA CARE!

Click this link to get started:

https://www.subscribepage.com/life-giving-dementia-care-checklists

Dedication

This effort is dedicated to my mother, Lois Virginia Bridgeman Noland, aka Nana. She and my dad taught me to reach for my dreams; that I was only limited by my effort. This mindset serves you well when authoring a book. There can be so many obstacles. Perseverance is key, along with confidence that this can really happen. She was inspiration for this work. Her incredible positivity, never give up attitude, and complete, unconditional love gave me the direction and strength to pursue this dream. She inspired me every day. I love and miss her.

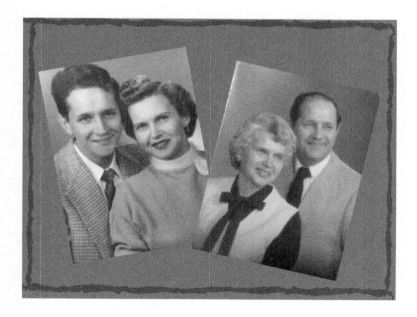

Contents

Introduction

"Weeds are flowers too, once you get to know them."
- Winnie the Pooh

My name is Toni, and I'm a dementia caregiver. Once you're a caregiver, you're always a caregiver. The caregiving experience changes you that much.

I'm also a Winnie the Pooh fan. He inspires me, how he pauses to think, think, think, and then says exactly the right thing, or asks the perfect question—the one that's right in front of the grownups' faces, but they can't, or won't, see it.

This quote about weeds and flowers is perfect. It says the obvious, with a simple twist. It's the perfect summation of the message in these pages.

Dementia caregiving feels like living in the weeds; like those pesky dandelions that are here today, gone tomorrow, then back again in a week with a dozen fuzzy, white cousins. They endlessly tease us with temporary beauty.

But there's another perspective. Pooh knows this, and so does every child who sees a dandelion. Catch their joy, running barefoot through a field of golden yellow. See their wonder when surrounded by fluffy white puffballs that disappear in the wind, floating to everywhere, and to nowhere.

With the right perspective, weeds are wondrous.

The Bucket List

Do you have a Bucket List? I do. It includes creative efforts like make a stained-glass window and a queen size quilt. I want to take a Broadway play tour and go to Hawaii, to lose weight and have grandchildren. I'd like to audit Ivy League online classes and publish a children's book. I intentionally included lots of interesting, mind-stretching goals over the years.

Being a dementia caregiver was nowhere on my list.

From the summer of 2013 until the spring of 2016, that is exactly what I was—primary caregiver for my mom (referred to as Nana in these pages), diagnosed with the Alzheimer's form of dementia. Her diagnosis marked the first of many rounds of the grief process for me during her illness. I believed her doctors, but I didn't accept it for months. Nana never, ever, believed or accepted it. "Those doctors are crazy!" she said.

Things make it onto your bucket list because you want them there. You eagerly anticipate and plan each experience. You may take classes or read books, do research, and budget for the cost. You prepare.

Becoming caregiver for a loved one is not generally something you prepare to do. Rather, it falls into your lap. Even though I'm an only child and knew I would eventually need to care for my parents, it never occurred to me to prepare. No research, no reading. Not even the occasional article or news story.

I don't want to sound cliché, but if you're new at this caregiver gig, you simply don't know what you don't know.

Why Author a Book About Dementia?

I'm an overachiever by nature, so I worked hard at this new challenge. I made sure Nana followed the doctor's orders, got to her endless appointments, had at least one healthy meal available every day, and was as mentally stimulated as I could interest her in being. It took loads of time and energy, but I loved my mom and was determined to do my best. After all, she devoted her life to me, literally, and earned every ounce of love and respect I could muster. My role was to check off every box. The problem was my checklist was missing lots of boxes.

Despite my best efforts, I made mistakes. So. Many. Mistakes. My mean words, misunderstanding her behaviors, and my fits of impatience took an emotional toll and hurt Nana. They became part of my *Regret List*, a list no one wants to claim.

Research tells us that, other than early-onset dementia, the highest risk factor to developing dementia is age.[1] Generally, from the mid-60's through our 80's, as our brain cells begin to die, they become *gunky*, to put it simply. Both my parents lived with dementia. Nana was medically diagnosed, but my dad refused to be tested, though we all knew he had it, too.

It seems, as with many diseases, I have a much higher risk of developing dementia because one of my parents had it. The fact both had it further increases my risk. Data shows that, if dementia affected your mother rather than your father . . . let's just say it's wise to prepare for a possible dementia diagnosis.[2]

Which brings me to the dual purpose of this book: preparation and encouragement.

You see, I expect my children will likely care for me if and when I need help. We generally like each other quite a bit. I have three sons, and at one time or another, they each have been momma's boys. There's no shame in that, as long as I don't interfere too much in their lives, and (let's be honest here) they don't mess too much with mine.

I'll be clear—I love my sons, so much. I know that they and their families will take care of me if my dementia time comes. It's because of that love that this book came about.

About a year after Nana died due to her dementia and its many complications, memories of that time started to replay in my mind. How I felt at different times during her illness and decisions I made or didn't make but should have. Plans we made together, and separately. The funny things that happened, the silliness, and the sadness we worked through. The pain of losing so much of her, yet gaining so much.

Through all of this, I kept returning to the same two undeniable facts: I made a lot of mistakes, and it took me far too long to learn to relax and go with the daily flow (which is just one more mistake).

Initially, my idea was to document the things I learned along the way in caring for my mom and share those with my boys. Things they should know so they don't repeat my mistakes, to hopefully help the journey be less stressful for them and maybe bring some joy. At least make it more memorable in a positive way. It was not, initially, a book. At best, it would be an exceptionally long letter.

Over time, I noticed an alarming number of friends and co-workers struggling to care for loved ones with dementia. I'm not exaggerating—the prevalence of this experience among my 45- to 60-year-old groupies was stunning.

As we commiserated, sharing notes and tears, I found that sharing my experiences helped them. The more open I was about my mistakes as well as successes, the more encouraged they were. I love to encourage people—I'm an Enneagram 3w2 (look it up).[3] Encouragement and seeing the silver lining are in my DNA.

Fast forward through lots of research, prayer, and a 20-year-old conviction that I was called to be a writer (don't ask why it took me 20 years to act on that). I realized I could kill two birds with one stone.

I'd author a book for my boys, to my boys, recording as much as I could about what they would need to know to take their absolute best care of me. Just lessons from me, to them. Sharing my failures and successes with Nana, teaching them they can grow through this journey, and how.

This same book would also serve my friends and co-workers . . . and you. Anyone who gets up one day to find they're faced with the necessity, the opportunity . . . the gift . . . of caring for their parent or a loved one through dementia. The principles are the same regardless of the terminal illness.

To Prepare and Encourage

This book is intended to encourage you. Part how-to guide, part memoir. Please don't be sad by any stories shared, or the images painted at times when maybe I'm a bit too brutally honest. If this disease comes to your loved one, to a friend . . . or to you personally someday . . . I pray these stories and lessons learned can give you comfort and guidance. I hope it gives a huge dose of encouragement that you can do this, and you will.

In this book, I use the term *dementia* because that was Nana's diagnosis. But this is an overarching word. Think of dementia as an umbrella with distinct types underneath, such as Alzheimer's, Vascular, Lewy Body, and others. If you read a reference to Alzheimer's, remember that it falls under the dementia umbrella.

Each chapter is designed to stand alone and be plucked out when you need it. I've included an executive summary closing each for those times when you simply have no time.

Also, in most chapters, you'll see sections in *italics*. These are written from the perspective of your dementia patient, telling you what they may be, or will be, experiencing, and helping you know how to react or what to do to help them. Sort of like being inside their head, as it were.

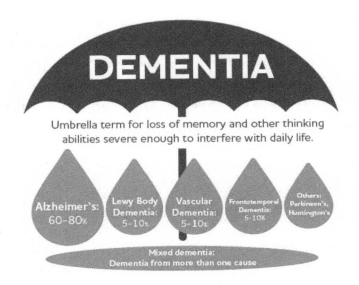

Honestly, I hope someday this book won't be necessary. I hope that dementia is something our great-greats had, back in the day. That cancer, Parkinson's, ALS, and so many other terminal illnesses will be eliminated.

My goal for you, dear reader, is simple. I want you to feel like you are sitting across the table from a good friend, drinking a cup of your favorite java or tea—to also have your loved one right there occasionally sharing a glimpse of the world from their point of view. All the fears, questions, emotions racing around your brain can be laid bare, and we can talk about them. I hope it feels like we're talking to you, sharing what we learned and how not to feel so lost or scared.

Because I've been there, I do know what you don't know. And I'm not afraid, or ashamed, to lay it all out so that your journey as a caregiver is as fulfilling as possible. So much joy is possible if that is your goal.

I want you to see what Pooh and I see—the weeds, they are flowers, too, once you get to know them.

Part I

The Early Stage

Chapter 1

How Do You Know
There's a Problem?

"The first step in solving a problem is recognizing there is one"
- AARON SORKIN

My Aunt Hollis lived in a 12' wide trailer. It was filled with colorful afghans and crochet dolls she bought at craft fairs in their small town or from the crafty neighbor who lived behind the raspberry bush fence. Visiting her was like strolling through a flea market or antique store. The smell of dusty knick-knacks and mismatched furniture blended into the scent of "old," that smell that reminds you of nursing homes. But her place felt like love to me, so I always looked forward to visiting.

Most of Nana's family lived in southern Illinois. Because of work schedules, we only made the trip to visit twice each year, usually around Memorial Day to put flowers on graves, and for the summer family reunion. It was during a May 2008 visit with Aunt Hollis that I first witnessed the warning signs of dementia.

I noticed she was a little crankier than usual. Aunt Hollis had been widowed, for the third time, about six months before. She was hard of hearing and always spoke loudly, with a backwoods drawl. That day she was louder and more animated than usual. I didn't think too much about it, though, since she was complaining about my cousins, which was always a loud affair.

What caught my attention was when she stopped talking. The quiet. That just never happened. I walked into the kitchen to find her crying. Aunt Hollis always had a hankie because of her sinus issues; she never held one because she was crying. Yet, there she sat, sobbing almost uncontrollably.

I was stunned. Comforting her, I asked why the tears. She had no clue.

This continued for a while that day and repeated several times during our visit. Every time, I tried to help. She never seemed to realize this was a repeating pattern. She vigorously denied it. "Yore jes gittin oldtimers! You better git yourself to the doctor," she barked at me. It was unexpected behavior, even for her. My uncle told us the doctor diagnosed dementia.

The Mayo Clinic[4] and AARP[5] websites list the early warning signs of dementia. There's a fine line between the normal cognitive decline that begins in our fifties and the time behaviors progress into the yellow area of "concerning." It's one thing to fumble to come up with my favorite actor's name. It's another if I put the milk in the pantry, on purpose. That type of thing. Unexpected changes in memory, in personality, making uncharacteristic choices or comments, experiencing confusion that is unwarranted—all of these might be big yellow caution signs. To be prepared and equipped to spot the signs of dementia, you need to educate yourself, and you'll need to know your loved one well enough to spot the changes.

It's Kind of Like Driving Without a Roadmap

Generally speaking, you'll need to watch for a decline in my ability to perform daily functions, to drive safely, to pay bills, if I am losing track of sequences like showering before I get dressed instead of after. You will see changes in my "three B's": behavior, body, and brain. I may not admit it, but I am noticing these things, and I'm scared.

Most books give disease or care information in general terms. Yes, there are commonalities among all dementia patients. But in reality, the disease looks a little different for every person. We are each created uniquely, and dementia manifests like that—uniquely, one person at a time. How can I describe this?

Imagine that you are driving to the Rocky Mountains to hike. You know you're headed to Estes Park and it will take about 20 hours, so you should get there tomorrow afternoon, assuming an overnight stay in Kansas City. A good map is all you need, right?

But as you near the Colorado border, trivial things start to derail your plans. Nothing major, at first. You're hungry, but reaching for the cooler in the back seat, you find the spare one that stores extra ice packs. Not the one packed with the turkey and provolone sandwiches on pretzel buns you made. And Kettle chips. Nope. Nothing there. Well, no biggie. You can get some grub in the next town.

You check your phone to see how far it is to the nearest town, but your phone is dead. You reach for the charger—you brought the wrong charger. Also, normally not a huge problem. You can buy one down the road.

Except there seems to be a big accident up ahead, and the traffic is stopped. Not slowed, but a complete standstill. You're getting hungrier and realize it's time for your meds, which require food. You don't have any food, not even a bag of Skittles.

But good news. Police are diverting traffic. You're finally moving. Unfortunately, there aren't detour signs, and the cars ahead of you are going all different directions on the roads so you can't reliably follow them to civilization. You don't have access to the phone GPS since your phone is dead, and your car doesn't have GPS to guide you. The old, paper map in the glovebox got wet from the hand sanitizer that leaked, so, now you don't even have that. Surely, you'll get to a town soon, though. Follow the sunset, right?

And, of course, the gas gauge starts to hit red territory and beep. Who thought it was smart to space gas stations 100 miles apart out west? At this point, you don't know where you are, how you got there, where you are trying to go, how long it will take, or if you or the car will make it.

If you only had a map. And someone knowledgeable to navigate.

Being a dementia caregiver is like this. You may have a map that shows beginning and ending points, with some key detours marked along the way. But there's no crystal ball foretelling all these points because the journey is uniquely yours, different from everyone else's.

We all know little problems can quickly become big messes. The key to successfully managing most situations is having a good plan and great co-pilot—having a navigator who knows you, the driver, well enough to predict the little things that might be overlooked, forgotten, or left behind. A helper who knows the road, or how to find help when it's needed. You need someone who understands the road behind and ahead well enough to recognize coming dangers.

This is where you fit in. I'll need you to help me create a plan. You'll need to spend time with me to know what is normal and what is not. Sometimes that might mean spending time apart so changes are more obvious. I need you to be my co-pilot, and eventually, my driver. I may not ask for this help, or in some ways feel I need it. But I do and will count on you to watch, anticipate my needs, and lovingly walk us forward.

If It Looks Like a Duck . . . Behavior Signs

Let's dive a little into the technical information about Dementia. You can read the medical causes and jargon on your own—I have included resources in the appendix. My goal here is to teach what you should know so we can walk through this together, with dignity for me and sanity for you.

There are two schools of thought about how the disease progresses: the 3-stage model, and the 7-stage model. I will focus on the 3-stage model:[6] Early, Middle, and Late. Not terribly original, but it's simple and easy to remember (no pun intended). I'll address middle and late stages in the next sections, and we'll touch on the 7-stage model in Chapter 6.

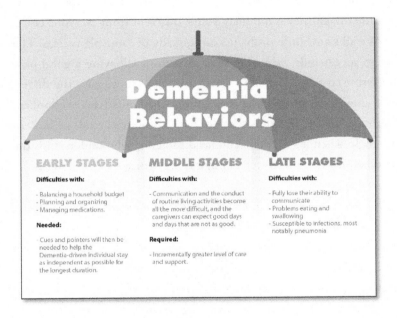

EARLY STAGES

Difficulties with:

- Balancing a household budget
- Planning and organizing
- Managing medications.

Needed:

Cues and pointers will then be needed to help the Dementia-driven individual stay as independent as possible for the longest duration.

MIDDLE STAGES

Difficulties with:

- Communication and the conduct of routine living activities become all the more difficult, and the caregivers can expect good days and days that are not as good.

Required:

- Incrementally greater level of care and support.

LATE STAGES

Difficulties with:

- Fully lose their ability to communicate
- Problems eating and swallowing
- Susceptible to infections, most notably pneumonia

The early stage of my disease will generally be milder in impact. Old age "normal" will begin to intensify and interfere with my daily living. You will notice me forgetting more often and more intensely. My frustration at this will cause me to become cranky and argumentative, at times. This can cause you extreme distress if you're not prepared for it. Just remember, I may be in denial and most certainly will be frustrated and afraid.

My parents were serial accusers, looking for and generally finding ways the other was exhibiting "Oldtimers," as they put it. Since they lived with my family for 12 years or so, it could become irritating. But mostly we found it to be harmless. I could tell that their behavior was changing, especially Nana's.

She was always buying me something. That's the "curse" of being an only child—getting near constant gifts, whether you like what is bought or not. She called me into her room one evening after dinner, unusually excited, and pointed to a large box in the corner. "I got you something I know you'll love!" That was my clue to be super animated in my surprise, whatever it was.

I opened a heavy cardboard box holding four other boxes. The larger ones held an early generation Instant Pot. It looked like a pressure cooker to me, which I already owned. I had no idea what it actually was.

Apparently, Nana had seen a commercial on TV and thought this would be perfect to save me time. She always felt like I worked too much, and too hard, at my career and could use help cooking for the seven of us. As a bonus, this purchase included a cookbook, a steamer insert, a rubberized spoon, and a ladle . . . and a second Instant Pot. We didn't need two, but the exclusive offer included a buy-one-get-one offer, so she figured, why not? We can give it away as a gift. What she didn't realize was that she paid $85 in shipping for that "free" pot. From Georgia. BOGO—not quite.

Buying gifts for no reason was not unusual for her, regardless of the cost. Her generosity did more for her than for the recipient. Three days later, a second identical shipment arrived. No kidding.

When I called the company to share their error and arrange the return, they said she had placed two separate orders. Nana argued with me about it, but it was clear she did this. She didn't have a clue, but I had evidence, not just from the supplier.

You see, she kept these notepads on the nightstand, her constant brain dump. All day, as she watched soaps and courtroom reality shows, she would make notes on the pad of interesting information, new things she learned and wanted to tell me, and things she wanted to buy. If she did make a purchase, she'd record the date, cost, confirmation number, and so forth. These daily journals of sorts eventually became my roadmap to her mind's failure. They showed me where she had been, where she was going, and what she was thinking so I could redirect her and be prepared. Between the notepad and the supplier receipts, I knew exactly what she'd been up to.

My first reaction to all this was frustration that she was arguing with me about it, which then turned to anger because she was wasting money they simply did not have. That blew over, though, and we both moved on, chalking it up to old age forgetfulness. Until it happened again. And again.

I started checking in on her more frequently, often finding her on hold with some salesman. My dad was no help at all, as he simply didn't have the gumption to tell her no. I eventually started taking her credit cards away on the sly one at a time, saying she must have lost it. The fact she actually believed that was one more indication there was trouble in River City.

One day she tried to order a necklace for me and couldn't find her VISA. As usual, I said she must have lost it. She paused and replied, "Well, ok," and moved on. She didn't care at all. Who was this woman, and where was my mother? That was when I realized that Papaw might have some memory issues, but Nana was the one with real problems brewing. I knew we needed to talk to the doctor.

Weebles Wobble . . . Body Signs

Physical changes were easier to notice. She would become dizzy and lose her balance, but she always explained this as fatigue or she hadn't eaten enough. But I could tell there was a problem. I also saw her lose track of sequences when she was cooking. She'd search for a pan, a spoon, a fork, or a ladle. Then, she'd look for a pan again though she already had one. She would forget her next steps. This had to be frustrating for her. It was completely unnerving for me, and I couldn't ignore it. So, I decided to mention this at her next medical appointment.

I talked to both her primary care physician and her vascular doc. Both offered the same suggestion—Physical Therapy. Nana thought this was ridiculous. After all, she had been standing on her feet, working, until the age of 80. In her mind, she was strong, healthy, and not injured, so she certainly didn't need physical therapy. But she'd do anything to make me happy, so she agreed to give it a shot.

Her therapist, Ben, was truly kind and genuinely wanted to help. His visits became her twice-weekly personal challenge, and after some benign complaints, she usually rose to the occasion. He would ask her to do leg lifts or move her arms around. She would proudly walk laps around the living room. When he asked her to perform an activity, she did a few extra reps, with an indignant enthusiasm, basically announcing, "See I can do these things. I don't need physical therapy!"

Attitude aside, her balance and strength improved, and after a few weeks, it was decided she could continue exercises on her own. Which surprisingly she did, even being proud of herself. The lesson learned here can be summed up with this slightly altered idiom: Catch me once, shame on you, catch me twice, shame on me. Application? Don't ever allow excuses for the unusual, eventually dangerous, physical changes you see.

Here's a quick rundown of some of the most frequent changes you might catch me doing in this early stage or that may signal problems ahead.[7]

- *Change in my gait*
- *Loss of balance*
- *Worsening posture*
- *Pacing for no apparent reason—showing restlessness*
- *Worsening grip, dropping things*
- *Extreme change in my sleep patterns*

I will probably offer an excuse for all of them. But don't be fooled. I may not have a dementia diagnosis, yet, but something is wrong. Find a way to get me checked out.

The Record's Stuck . . . Brain Signs

The third area of change is my brain—mental slip-ups. Forgetfulness, repetition, loss of logic, and depression to name a few. These signs might be the trickiest to notice because some of this is natural as I age. It's important for you to pay close attention to what I say and do. To connect the dots. I will need you to see the things I can't and won't.

Let me illustrate this. In our home, Nana and Papaw basically owned the main floor. Master suite, bathroom, laundry, kitchen, living room—everything they needed was on that level. Except us. We spent most of our time upstairs since it was 1,500 square feet of loft living area, bedrooms, and two full baths. Everything we needed except the kitchen and laundry. For most of 12 years sharing our home, if she needed something or had a question, Nana would yell my name up the stairs or call my cell phone. This was grating at times, but it worked.

16

In 2014, she began to do this multiple times each evening. Ridiculous numbers—ten, fifteen, or more times yelling my name or her questions up the stairs when I was literally 10 feet away. Once I got to her room, she would ask the same questions every time, denying that we had just talked about them.

Becoming angry and impatient with her was one of my first, epic fails during her illness. I would foolishly try to argue with her when she would do this, eventually ignoring her when she called my name. Yes, I still feel awful about that. How could I have been so unaware? So silly? So uncaring? Mainly because I was ignorant about dementia and unprepared for what life was becoming; because I didn't learn to change my expectations until it was nearly too late.

Summary Points

- Make sure you watch well enough to spot changes that might signal cognitive illness; know the signs.

- You'll need to prepare to provide care—learn about this illness, help to plan, and be ready to guide.

- Watch for changes in the "three B's": behavior, body, and brain; keep a journal of what you see.

- Don't make assumptions—it may simply be old age. But if concerns are there, talk to the medical team.

Once you know there is a problem, help me get evaluated. That's the first step on our journey to manage my mental decline and all the challenges that come with dementia. This might not be easy, and I may fight you. Don't give up—we can build a team to help.

Chapter 2

Doctors and Testing and Planning, Oh My!

"You don't have to see the whole staircase, just take the first step."
- MARTIN LUTHER KING, JR.

The running joke in our home, while all seven of us lived together, involved my dad (Papaw) and "Oldtimers." The conversation would go something like this.

My dad would wander, clearly looking for something.

Nana would bark, "Bruce, what in the sam hill are you doing?"

"I'm trying to find my keys!" Papaw would bark right back. "Leave me alone!"

"I'm gonna take you to get one of them Oldtimers tests at the doctor. That's what's wrong—you've got Oldtimers, dad-gum-it!"

This exchange would recycle often. One day, the tables turned, and my dad came to me wondering if Nana should be tested. We both saw the signs—signs that she was struggling in many ways, but always had excuses.

Over the next few days, we discussed our next steps. Nana was proud and fiercely independent. Getting her to agree to a doctor's visit and cognitive testing would not happen easily, if at all.

It was decided I would assume management of her medical care to begin this process. Papaw was struggling to manage his own health, so my husband had begun helping him. Nana's number one goal in life was to make me happy, so we could use that to convince her to be evaluated.

Step 1: Choosing a Doctor

Your first step will be to talk with my primary care physician (PCP). Because of health care privacy laws, they probably won't talk with you. If Dad is able and available, he should already be authorized to get my medical information and can give you authorization, too, when you need it. If he's not available, do what's needed to get my direct permission for the PCP to discuss my medical care. In short, trick me if you have to.

Schedule a first meet-and-greet appointment to talk alone with my PCP. You may have to pay for this, but it's important to choose the right doctor for us, to discuss what you see and what should be done next. Some PCPs will do an evaluation themselves; others might refer you to a neurologist or other specialist.

After talking with Nana's PCP, I decided to consult a gerontologist for evaluation. The excuse I offered for adding yet another doctor to her village was this—she had so many physicians, and they needed to coordinate to keep her healthy. If she wanted me to help her, I needed one doctor to oversee everyone. We decided that would be her gerontologist, a doctor who specialized in seniors like Nana. Since doing this would ultimately help me, she was happy to go.

That worked like a charm, and she was eager to prove she "wasn't like all those other old women." I did not warn her she would take a driving ability assessment that could ultimately wrest those precious car keys from her bony, work-scarred fingers.

If you decide to take me to a specialist, I recommend you get referrals from the PCP, friends, online—wherever you can get reliable information. You'll be attached at the hip to this doctor, so make sure you like and trust them. Prepare a list of questions like these to interview them in your first one-on-one appointment.

- *What is their philosophy on patient care?*
- *What is your feeling about their bedside manner, and do you think their personality will mesh well with mine, and yours?*
- *How will they support us down the road?*
- *Can they be readily reached when needed?*
- *Will they stick with us to the end?*

Step 2: Studying for This Test Is Not Cheating

Getting reliable results on any test requires a basic understanding of what is being evaluated and how it will be administered. A dementia evaluation is like this. Your loved one will need to be prepared, and cooperative, to get reliable results and an accurate evaluation.

To that end, there are steps you should take before the evaluation appointment to prepare.

- Ask the physician for information about the test and process and review it before the appointment.
- Review reference information from the Alzheimer's Association (your new best friend).
- You probably know someone(s) who has gone through this or has relatable experiences. Contact them. I'm sure they'll be eager to share their experience.
- Let the PCP know which doctor we're visiting, and when, so medical records can be shared.

- Plan a special treat for after the appointment. Your loved one will be tired, confused, and who knows, maybe even angry or frustrated. Be ready for this. Something fun will help distract you both.

Because I'll be seeing a new doctor, it will seem natural that I would be tested. This is a wonderful opportunity to ease any of my fears and suspicions. You will already have reviewed testing materials, so talk with me about some of the tests that I'll take. Help me understand that I should do my best to respond well even though the questions might seem silly to me.

A word of warning here: Watch carefully to be sure I am not intentionally giving false answers. This might seem unlikely since I am, after all, being tested for cognitive decline. How could I be sharp enough to figure that out? Well, believe me, I can be.

Nana did this during her evaluation, or at least claimed she was "faking it" for fun after we pointed out that she did not correctly know the current season, or month, among other errors. It was challenging at times to know for sure if she was serious or playing games. The doctor ended up giving her a couple of different question sets to be sure.

Just remember, preparing ahead of time will make this key appointment go much more smoothly and supply better results.

Step 3: Testing 'R Us

I can hear Nana complaining in my head, "It ain't multiple choice, that's for sure." Cognitive evaluation is intentionally sneaky, to some degree. After all, who honestly wants to take a test like this, or worse, fail it? You should do your own research on the latest evaluation techniques. The Alzheimer's Association publishes an online test toolkit that explains it well.[8] This is where you should begin.

> *In general, the evaluator will ask questions to know me better. They'll give me some information, like a person's name and specific address, and ask me to repeat it in a few minutes. They might ask simple things like what season it is, or month, who our current president is, or my address.*
>
> *They might show me a picture of a clock with hands and ask me the time. We'll discuss current events—do I know any, and what can I explain. Another typical exercise is to give me a brief list of common, unrelated words, maybe three to four, and then ask me to recall them in two to three minutes. Apple, penny, table.*

As with all good tests, patients earn, or lose, points based on their responses. Points are given for remembering, correctly; fewer points are earned if help is needed. Points for how long it takes to respond, and no points if they appear lost. Some assessments may involve evaluating physical skills, like the driving test.

Of course, we did not tell Nana she was taking a driving assessment. She would have refused. Nothing was ever going to stop her from driving—to her that car was everything. It was her independence, and therefore, her self-worth. She did fail the test, though, twice (they readministered it since she insisted the first set of results were wrong), and she forever referred to the evaluating doctor as "that crazy doctor who took my keys!"

How she failed was interesting. She lost points for two reasons. First, her decision-making was poor. For example, she saw a car pulling out in front of her. Instead of slowing, or stopping, she ran into them because "it was their fault—they pulled out in front of me, the dummy!"

But the main reason she failed was due to horrible response time.

Using a driving simulator machine, she ran into everything and everybody because it took her so long to see the situation, assess her options, make a choice, and then get her body to act. Funny, we forget how many steps, decisions, are involved in driving. It becomes automatic for us.

She refused to accept the driving test results. Nana was great at excuses. The doctor was crazy. The machine was broken. Trees were in the way, and no one in their "right mind" could avoid crashing on that test. "They just want to take my car. Well I won't let them!" I rarely saw her as angry and defiant. What were we in for when we got her full dementia test results?

Step 4: Results Come in Different Shapes and Sizes

I'll be honest—even if in your heart of hearts, you know I have dementia, you will be anxious to hear the results. This diagnosis is just like having your first child—it changes everything and rocks your world. And it will rock mine. You may have prepared for the doctor visit and studied for the evaluation tests. You may be expecting a dementia diagnosis. But you can't truly be prepared for it.

Your physician will talk alone with you to understand what you have seen, your primary concerns, and why you choose to evaluate now. Bring your notes, journal, or whatever you've used to track worrisome behaviors. This will save you time, and money, and will become part of their evaluation and diagnosis.

The doctor will add more points toward my testing total based on your comments about how I manage at home. Do I remember the steps to make my bed? Do I turn off the stove or leave the water running? Do my clothes match, assuming they did before (quiet in the peanut gallery, please), or is there a change in my appearance? All the things you've been tracking.

The examiner may be able to supply a diagnosis right then. For some people, diagnosis might take up to a year. So much depends on the appointment results. During this one-on-one time, ask when we will get test results and a diagnosis and how you will receive them. Who will receive them—you, the patient, or both? Find out the next steps medically, like follow up appointments, visits with other related specialists, or safety modifications needed at home. There are many things to consider, and it may seem overwhelming. Adopt this mantra: if you prepare well, you can do much better than simply cope. You can grow as a person, and your relationship with your loved one can thrive.

Step 5: Follow the Yellow Brick Road

If they "pass" the evaluation and don't receive a dementia diagnosis, you at least have baseline data for future comparison. After all, there are several medical conditions that can mimic dementia such as vascular disease or ageing itself. Keep in mind that having early cognitive results is a huge benefit—don't consider it time wasted.

With any diagnosis, you should get a second opinion.[9] There are other factors that could manifest dementia-like symptoms. Think about their overall situation. If any of these are factors, another perspective would be helpful.

- Nutritional imbalance
- Toxins or inflammation
- Prescription meds side effects
- Stress from life changes
- Hormonal issues
- Sleeping or breathing issues, hearing loss
- Physical inactivity, low mental or social stimulation, or frequent urinary tract infections

For discussion, let's assume your loved one received a diagnosis of dementia, maybe even the most common form of dementia—Alzheimer's.

Ideally, dementia would be their only physical issue. Unfortunately, that's highly unlikely. According to the U.S. Department of Health and Human Services, more than 5 million Americans live with dementia.[10] It's a disease that requires elevated levels of medical care and usually leads to a need for long-term services and supports. Most people with dementia live with additional chronic medical conditions such as diabetes, hypertension, or congestive heart failure. Health care costs will be higher with dementia than for folks with the same conditions that aren't also cognitively impaired. Such patients are more likely to be hospitalized or need home health or nursing home care. Brain issues complicate everything.

In short, make sure to be familiar with ALL my ailments, and of our family medical history, so you can be on the lookout for other warning signs and best manage my needs and costs. You'll need to do more research. To work with me, there are a lot of pieces to the medical puzzle. I also deal with heart, kidney, vascular, and thyroid disease along with Osteoporosis and COPD. Papaw had heart and kidney disease, diabetes, and COPD. All of these can contribute to cognitive decline and complicate my treatment. This is why it is so important for you to know my history, get my buy-in for you to help, and coordinate my medical care. Don't just take over and treat me like a child, even if I begin to act like one.

Their diagnosing physician should provide current information and resources. Nana's gerontologist had a delightful woman on staff, Jenny, who met with me during our results appointment. We discussed how I was dealing with this, what Nana's medical care would look like moving forward, how their office could help, and other available resources. She was extremely helpful.

Read the information, learn what to do, sooner rather than later. Visit the organization websites they direct you to. Call them, review their resources. Believe me—this is time well spent. You will use most of this information at some point.

You'll be directed to arrange future medical appointments. Don't be surprised if the follow-up visit with your diagnosing physician is not for another year. If their evaluation is borderline, or shows very early signs of dementia, they may recommend you give the disease time to manifest before making many changes. The medical staff may schedule some of the other initial visits for you. Ask about this as it will save you a lot of time if they do. Make sure you fully understand who you will see, why, and what care they will provide. The number of doctors can quickly become unmanageable, and there may be a domino effect.

During her evaluation, Nana's doctor suspected she might also have Osteoporosis. They scheduled an appointment with an endocrinologist, who then suspected her thyroid might be contributing to bone density loss. He referred her to an ear, nose, and throat specialist, so now we had three new doctors. The ENT eventually removed 75% of her thyroid, which did indeed improve her Osteoporosis. But see how quickly medical care can cascade into a hot mess if not managed well?

To avoid disaster, develop a system to track my appointments, doctors, their locations, purpose, and results—all the typical data. Use your phone calendar, set up a separate calendar just for my appointments, or use a journal (physical or online). There are many options, so pick one that works for you and is online so you can share it with others who can help in my care. It will help me feel some amount of control if I also have a calendar with my appointments. You'll need to remind me anyway, but seeing the calendar will comfort me.

I didn't track Nana's appointments well at first. Why would I ever lose track of something simple like a few doctor appointments? But after getting some dates mixed up and showing up at the wrong address, I saw the error of my ways and started using a Nana dedicated phone calendar. That one step became my lifesaver.

Summary Points

- Pick a physician to do the evaluation.

- Prepare both of you for the visit—to know who, what, where, why, and when.

- Prepare for the evaluation and testing.

- Study the evaluation results and do your homework on the next steps—should we get a second opinion?

- Start your medical follow-up visits by setting up your tracking process.

Following these steps will help you deal with a dementia diagnosis more effectively. You can simplify the "dos and don'ts" of being a dementia caregiver; it's a matter of perspective and preparation.

Chapter 3

Responding to a
Dementia Diagnosis

"If you expect nothing, you can never be disappointed."
– TONYA HURLEY

Dictionary.com defines the word cope as "to face and deal with responsibilities, problems, or difficulties, especially successfully or in a calm or adequate manner."[11] I find this humorous—the definition itself stresses me out. I'm not sure "calm and adequate" is possible for a dementia caregiver. At least not without lots of practice and planning.

Your instinct will be to find ways to personally cope. As needs increase, so will your successes, failures . . . and frustration. You'll be tired, confused, angry, encouraged, discouraged, tired again.

If your goal is just to cope, you are setting the bar too low. Let me explain.

You Can Learn Something from Everything

The toddler and teen years are among the most difficult of any parent's experience. The "terrible twos" and "hormonal teen" years are not just myths. They are very real. Veteran parents tried to help me through that time by sharing their sage advice. They would whisper, "this, too, shall pass, dear," or "don't worry—they'll be grown and gone before you know it." In other words, suffer through it until it eventually ends.

Yes, there were days when I adored my kids . . . but didn't like them all that much. Times when, driving to the grocery, I wondered what might happen if I continued to the west coast. I never did that, and I never would. The point is the sense of helplessness you feel at times can be suffocating if left unchecked. Something has to give.

Over the course of parenting three boys, I realized the "suffer through it" advice I received did hold one element of truth—at some point the experience will end. But that counsel failed by encouraging me to emotionally check out of that time in my life. To use the "grin and bear it" approach. That is so unfortunate.

You see, there is something truly special, once in a lifetime, which happens when children are 2, or 12 . . . or 16 years old. You should savor those times, when bonds are strengthened, not rush through. That was when I learned the most about their strengths and fears. They learned my love was unconditional, that I would love them no matter what they said or did. Through normal trial and error, we learned to be creative in our activities, patient in our conversations, and compassionate in our arguments.

This is exactly the perspective you should adopt as a dementia caregiver. Coping is essentially a self-centered approach, in my experience. It's all about you and getting through the challenge of the day in one piece. It ignores your loved one and the many blessings found by simply living in the moment.

This begs the question—how do you change your perspective, practically speaking? You do so by lowering your expectations for just about everything related to your loved one.

That might sound counterintuitive, but it works. Unfortunately, it took me two years to figure this out. I wish I could say my realization was a moment of epiphany, but in reality, it was an exasperated, last-ditch effort at survival. It got to the point I couldn't take Nana's constant inconsistencies anymore. When I finally gave up and decided to ditch all my expectations of her, I felt free for the first time since her diagnosis.

Of course, there are some expectations that you should keep. You should expect my reactions to be inconsistent. I may laugh or cry at odd or inappropriate times, argue about things I used to accept, or even switch sides on key cultural or political topics. Our roles may reverse in lots of ways, eventually with you becoming more like the parent and me more like the child. This is part of my disease and nothing to fear.

Dementia Caregiver Dos and Don'ts

No matter which stage of the illness you are experiencing, work hard to follow some key "Dos and Don'ts." It can move the experience dial from awful to precious in many ways. Later chapters will flesh out more details, but here's a list to get started.

The Dos . . .

- **DO pay close attention to what they do and say**. I know— I've already said this. But it bears repeating. This is key to you not just surviving but actually growing together.

- **DO keep a journal or digital record**—Anything where you can note what you observe or about interactions. Here's a spreadsheet example.

DATE	TIME	WHO	WHAT	MOOD	OUTCOME	NOTES
4/15/2020	8:30 a.m.	Bob & Mom	Breakfast	Quiet	Chatted, kept it light	3rd time this week Mom was quiet-work to get her talking

- **DO ask them questions to track how they're doing**. But please be patient and understand if they can't remember anything recent. You might need to be creative in how you ask to trigger memories. They can't help being forgetful, and you may even have to sift through their words to sort out fact from fiction. Remember it's not intentional.

- **DO cultivate a keen sense of humor**. Caregiving is not for the faint of heart. Just like you caused your parents some worried, sleepless nights, it can be terribly stressful to figure out what they'll be thinking or truly how they're doing. That's when your sense of humor can carry you through. And don't be surprised if their sense of humor changes, perhaps becoming a bit bawdier compared to pre-diagnosis. You'll probably find that more than amusing.

- **DO expect their personality to change**. I must admit, the unknown aspect of this was scary. It's not unusual for dementia patients to completely flip their personality, doing a 180° switch. Nana did this. She was a remarkable woman, and a fierce advocate, but she could be rather negative and was as stubborn as an ox. She was especially critical of certain people, but a staunch defender of others, and we never understood why she chose one over the other. Conversation in her later years could be downright tedious, often baffling, and at times disheartening.

Within a year of diagnosis, Nana became a real sweetheart, truly kind to everyone, complimentary, and grateful. Her prior negativity and critical nature vanished. It was amazing to experience and a blessing I can never adequately describe. Without that metamorphosis, I'm not sure how I could have provided her with the loving care she deserved.

That's also why I'm so afraid of this change for myself, should I develop dementia. Right now, I'm normally even tempered, generally kind, and can be pretty funny. Folks say I'm an encourager. Like everyone, I have my bad days, but what happens if my personality flips, and I become some mean, awful creature? A "dad-gummed hellcat" as Nana used to say. It's my worst nightmare. How can anyone care for me if I fight them every step of the way and make it miserable? I pray consistently that my frontal lobe behavior and memory function stays "un-gooed" as long as possible.

- **DO encourage them, and be sure to encourage yourself.** They likely have been a competent person. But this will change. Try not to be shocked or afraid when this happens. They will need your strength and resolve to show them they are still okay; changes are just another adventure. Encourage them to do things a new way or to learn something new. They'll be able to do that, especially in the early stage. Encourage them to create something lovely. And remember to find encouragement for yourself to accept the new person you see daily. Help them remember the things they can, without condescension.

- **DO expect their physical and mental abilities to change.** I wish changes would be gradual, but they won't be. In my

34

experience, it's more like a slight decline interspersed with giant drops, and maybe an occasional hop upward. Changes don't happen with any predictability, or regularity, so it's best to simply be ready for anything.

- **DO grieve.** Yes, you will grieve when they die. But a unique part of dealing with any terminal illness, especially dementia, is that multiple milestones occur during the journey. It's okay to grieve when they're diagnosed, as they start to exhibit major memory loss, or yet again when you have to plan the funeral or estate disposition. They need to grieve too, early on. Lean on each other.

The Don'ts . . .

- **DON'T patronize them.** This will be tricky, because at times they act or react like a child. You'll be tempted to lash out or slip into parent mode. I promise you—you will regret it if you do. Nana has been gone for years, and I still cringe at some of my snippy responses to her comments. Remember, their words will not necessarily be trustworthy, so you need to be the adult in the room.

- **DON'T be demeaning.** They struggle enough with fear, feelings of inadequacy, and confusion—actions they can't help. Nana would leave notes for me by the stove. I'd take the note, and before long, another note would appear. She couldn't remember she already left one. To get her to stop (which wasn't going to happen, anyway) and prove to her she kept leaving the same note, I would bring them all to her in a stack. The result was I was angry, and she would cry. I did that, seriously. An epic fail on my part.

- **DON'T argue with them**. That is such a waste of your time and energy. You can't win an argument with someone who has little logical ability. Make note of what they say, then agree, but take whatever action is needed. Nana was absolutely convinced that she still could drive. It didn't help that the Bureau of Motor Vehicles renewed her license. Even though I asked him not to, my dad took her to the branch, she passed her eye exam, and they handed her a shiny, new license. At that point, the doctor had already tested her driving ability, diagnosed Dementia, and I had taken her car keys. But how could the BMV know that? Since there is no "dementia registry" for them to cross-reference, they trust the family to not bring the patient in to get a license. I admit I argued with her for months about not driving, trying to use logic, replaying events—anything I thought might convince her. To what end? She never accepted the loss of freedom those car keys represented or the hit to her independent streak. I should not have argued—it often brought her to tears. Trust me, you don't want to see that.

- **DON'T say you already told them something**, maybe even multiple times in a day, and that they forgot. It will make them feel "less than." Less than an adult. Less than your parent. Less than competent. Less than worthy. Simply tell them again. Write it on a Post-it and put it on their wall or by the bed or chair. Find ways to answer respectfully and not lose your patience.

- **DON'T rush them**. They'll need more processing and transfer time. It'll take longer to dress, to go to the bathroom, to express themself. I'd get so impatient with

Nana at her medication time—it took her forever to swallow pills, and sometimes she would spit them back up. It was years later when I realized that her esophagus had narrowed, and she was easily choked.

Setting realistic expectations for me from the start will make life so much easier. It frees you to incorporate flexibility and creativity into our relationship. We'll be able to experience life in some fun, new ways, because eventually every day will be something new for me. Every experience will seem like it's the first time.

When I say that this is a new store, or the first time I've been down a street, or ask if you're wearing a new shirt (that I actually bought for you ten years ago), just smile and take pleasure in seeing my joy at experiencing something new.

I'll probably say this fifty times—frustration is your enemy, not dementia. Something else worth repeating . . . If your goal is just to cope, you are setting the bar too low. You may think, "Well, that's easy for you to say. *How*, in a practical way and on a daily basis, do I so dramatically change the ways I relate to them?" In a word—Community.

Summary Points

- Coping is self-centered and should not be your goal.

- Develop a perspective of finding the positives each day.

- Do encourage, pay attention to your loved one, track changes, and expect changes behaviorally, physically, and mentally. Be respectful. Grieve when you need to, for yourself and with them.

- Don't be patronizing, demeaning, impatient, or frustrated; arguing with them is a complete waste of time.

Once you've worked through your emotions about their diagnosis, you can begin to build a plan for how to practically deal with the realities of being a dementia caregiver. Your next step is to build a support village to help you move safely through your new normal.

Chapter 4

Build a Support Community

"Alone we can do so little; together we can do so much."
- HELEN KELLER

I have a friend in a quaint, small town. He owned an older, one-story home in the village that stopped serving his growing family. Property values had skyrocketed, and he noticed the inventory of larger homes was limited and pricey.

It seemed like the timing was good, so he decided to level his home and build a new one. Being an engineer, he took the pay-as-you-go route and served as his own project manager. In a few years, he completed a larger, beautiful new home on the same property that fit the town's architectural guidelines.

My point? To build, he had to destroy. This principal also applies to being a dementia caregiver.

Most of what you know about how I react, what I say or do, what I like to eat, or how to make me laugh will change over time. We'll need to interact differently. You'll learn new ways to help me. You'll learn that, in fact, I'm no longer self-sufficient and will need more of your help. To make room for the new me, you must throw out your old expectations.

Let me stress that setting realistic expectations for your loved one is vital. The key word is *realistic*. Initially, their ability to understand, to remember information, to listen carefully, and to make good decisions won't be too bad.

But their abilities will decline. Expect this, and adjust your thinking beforehand, not during or after. At that point, it may be too late to prevent or minimize your frustration. Alcoholics Anonymous says, "Expectations are Premeditated Resentments."[12] I have lived this journey and can say it's also true with dementia. You will eventually resent them unless you adjust your expectations.

Research can guide you, along with spending time with me. Other aspects of your life may have to go. You'll swap time with other family and friends to sit with me. You'll lose work and use PTO taking me to medical appointments. Time you spent watching TV may become time reading to me, looking at family videos or photos, or taking walks together. I may become your shadow as you work on hobbies. Is this a positive or not? Your perspective and expectations mean everything in our journey together.

Most tradeoffs can be positive if you set your expectations appropriately and keep a positive, hopeful perspective. I believe you can handle anything if you place your faith in Christ. I've lived this and can say with 100% certainty that it is true.

Who Should Be in Your Support Community?

Do you remember the rules of journalism? Every story should answer the questions who, what, where, when, and why. Building a support community is a lot like this.[13] You must be able to answer each of these questions to effectively surround yourself with the support you will need.

"One" Is the Loneliest Number

Why do you need a support community? You may initially believe this is all manageable. After all, you're intelligent, educated, resourceful. If you've known anyone who was a caregiver, or have read about caregiving, you probably picked up a lot of information. It's reasonable to think a few tools and friends should be enough to help you navigate whatever challenges will come along.

Let me say—you are dead wrong.

Consider my engineer/builder friend. He designed his new house; he estimated the cost and construction time. He lined up experts to fill in his experience and skill gaps. Certainly, he expected a few glitches, but overall, he felt prepared to complete the project.

Four YEARS later—yes, four—he moved into his new home. That was not the original plan. Unexpected events derailed his plans, and he needed more help and support than he ever imagined. In hindsight, which is always 20/20, he didn't just need a plumber, and a concrete guy, and a crane to lift the roof joists. He also needed friends to help insulate and pull wires on weekends, somebody to bring a home cooked meal, and a support team to lend a shoulder to lean on or let him vent about some sub-par contractor.

Instead of going solo, he needed a community to walk through the project with him, every step of the way. Doing that one step can save so much time, pain, and stress.

The Right Folks in the Right Seat

The "who" and "what" of support community members often go hand in hand. The first "who" group is people that are always there for you. Your spouse or close friends, for example. What they provide in support will be based on your relationship with them and their skills and abilities. You might pick some of these folks for specific tasks, but for the most part, you'll accept what they offer because they care about you and your loved one.

The second "who" group will be strangers, referred by the PCP or gerontologist. It's inevitable that your doctors will add others to your care community. This works if the care is coordinated; the medical team needs to know what each is doing for you. Nana went to a podiatrist regularly just to cut her toenails since they were too thick for us to cut. Medicare covered the cost, so why not? We didn't know to do this on our own—her vascular doctor referred us after examining her feet.

Especially in the later stages of my illness, you'll be the one adding others for support, like maybe a daycare, or in-home nurses. You may choose my visitors, lawyer, mortician, and financial folks, and guide my friend or church interactions. I may have some input, but mostly you'll direct who's included. I trust you to do what's best for me.

You should refer to the Alzheimer's Association or local council on ageing to get fresh guidance. I encourage you to also include a caregiver's support group for yourself.

I don't believe the number of people in your support community should be limited. One warning: you do have to be reasonable. No one needs five lawyers. But people will want to help, so let them. Don't be proud. Many won't know exactly how to help, so be prepared to be honest, and teach them. Ask for help. That will be a win-win-win for everyone.

Strangers and Google—Help Is Everywhere

Where will this support community come from? You might be surprised. In addition to folks that are intentionally added, others will be spontaneous. And sometimes the support will flow both directions.

About a year after Nana's diagnosis, I was shopping for her adult diapers. There were dozens of options, and I was still a rookie. An older man came near, and I quickly realized he was struggling with the many choices. I asked if I could help—what size was he looking for?

With teary eyes, he explained this was his first time shopping without his wife. She usually handled this during their weekly excursion. But this time, she couldn't join him. In fact, he probably would be doing all their shopping alone from now on.

We talked in the diaper aisle for nearly an hour, sharing stories about our loved one, the challenges, surprises, and disappointments. We were at different places in the journey, so it was encouraging to find someone who totally got it. He left, diapers in hand, being encouraged and feeling less alone.

I was encouraged from that encounter, too. I learned that my pain as an adult caring for my mother, while deep, was quite different from my new friend's pain as he watched the love of his life slip away. I learned that dementia progresses the same, but also a bit differently, for each person. And I learned that support could come out of the blue from unexpected sources.

Remember—post-diagnosis frustration is our real enemy, not the disease. The faster things change for me, the slower time may feel, as if it's in slow motion. And sometimes it may feel like you are in a time loop when I might decline and improve repeatedly. Like riding a roller coaster. Absolutely you should lean on others, and our support community, our "village," should be there right alongside you. This support is the key that gives us margin to build memories and grow through our journey.

Summary Points

- Make room for a new perspective—be open minded about your loved one and your journey together.

- Set realistic expectations—ditch idealism and preconceived notions.

- As you add people to your support community, ask and answer the five "W's": why, who, what, where, and when; ultimately, you choose them all, not the doctors.

- Encouragement can, and will, come unexpectedly—don't miss it by being distracted.

- Frustration can be a bigger enemy than the disease.

Building your support community may be the most crucial step. Surrounding yourself with those you trust, those who love you, and those who can fill in the gaps. It can be easy to distance yourself from your loved one and others to protect your emotions, your memories. Fight that. Amid all their changes, it is vital that you remember that things about them may change but they are still the same inside.

Chapter 5

Change Happens: Who Is This Person?

"I often hear people say that a person suffering from Alzheimer's is not the person they knew. I wonder to myself—Who are they then?"
- BOB DEMARCO

If the popular TV game show, *Family Feud*, used the question, "Name the top 10 signs someone has dementia," the number one response would likely be memory loss. This belief has long been popularized by media and entertainment. Yes, forgetfulness is one of the leading symptoms and one of the main losses in dementia, but it isn't the patient's greatest loss.

What, then, may be the biggest loss they can have from dementia? Their personality.[14]

Pay Attention, Please

My behavior and personality may change well before memory loss begins to affect my daily routine. Watch me closely, and don't ignore it when I'm not myself for longer than a few days. Dementia often first rears its ugly head in higher levels of anxiety, depression, or with my becoming withdrawn. I may hallucinate, become rude and uncaring, or be more confused and agitated later in the day (this is known as "sundowning").[15]

In hindsight, I can recognize this change in Nana. She was only a few years past a forced retirement, which she was still angry about and regularly threatened to sue her former employer. "How dare they force me to retire when I was only 80 years old," was her line of thinking. I can't say I blame her; she was still going strong.

When she started to be more agitated, down in the dumps, disagreeable, and withdrawn, I figured it was due to her job situation. Plus, her living siblings were in physical decline, and she worried about them. I also must admit we were in the middle of having kids in high school, newly married, or experiencing first-job pains, so life was remarkably busy. We weren't quite as engaged with her daily as we should have been.

In short, we didn't notice. I didn't notice. We didn't know what we didn't know.

We finally realized there was a problem when her memory loss became more obvious—when she made repeat purchases, asked the same questions ad nauseum, and forgot to take her pills. Eventually I was agitated enough to do some research. I wish I had known up front to look for behavior and personality changes. We might have started her treatment months, maybe years, earlier and avoided so much heartache for everyone.

The Physical Impact Can Vary Wildly

In addition to personality differences, my physical appearance will change. My steps may shorten, and I can lose muscle tone. My balance will become much less reliable. I ordered not one, but two, HurryCanes™ to steady myself (and because they looked so cool). Since my attention span will shorten, along with my memory, I may not dress as well, or remember to wear makeup or earrings each day. These are tasks that you can help me with to keep a sense of normalcy, and to keep my dignity. You should also notice if I take an interest in something new, because it can easily rise to the level of obsession.

My mom could be vain. She grew up in a large family of nine plus my grandfather (unfortunately, my grandmother died at age 38 shortly after giving birth to her eleventh child). Because she grew up poor, she insisted we wear the best, most colorful clothing we could find. This meant shopping at JC Penney department store every weekend. Seriously, we shopped—every weekend—for new clothes. Nana believed we should look like we just stepped out of a band box.[16] (You may need to look that one up, but let's just say we had to look good.)

Nana visited the hair salon weekly, like clockwork, but never showed any interest in painted nails until her eighties. Sometimes she commented about a celebrity's nails, and occasionally she would paint her toenails, letting the color wear off in a few weeks. Otherwise, she showed little interest.

During her dementia early stage, she started expressing an interest in nail polish.

Once while shopping in Costco, she bought a set of 10 polish bottles. I thought that was awesome, so we also bought polish remover.

A week later, she asked me to buy some nail polish. Thinking she simply forgot we just bought a bunch, I brought her the box we bought. Every one of the bottles was empty. When I asked where the polish went, she said they spilled and were all too old to use anyway. I picked up another set but started watching her more closely.

She painted her toenails two or three, sometimes four times each day. Her room smelled like a chemical factory from all the acetone polish remover. Every time she repainted, she'd insist that that color was weeks old and it was time for a change. Silly me would argue with her about it, to what end I don't know. Did it really matter all

47

that much? No. It made her happy. It would have been so much easier to simply distract her to move her along. It's amazingly easy to distract a dementia patient, and that's one of your most successful strategies to manage these obsessions.

My point is dementia patients undergo a multitude of changes. You should just get used to it. I noticed Nana's eyes were "dimming." They were just less . . . life-like, less like her, with no twinkle. You should understand something I didn't realize until several years after Nana's death.

No matter how different I look, how much my personality changes, or whether I call you by the correct name, or any name, I'm still Mom.

Still Mom

A rapidly fading photo lives on our refrigerator, held by a worn, red magnet frame. It was taken in December 2015 at Joy's House, an amazing adult daycare in Indianapolis. In it, Nana is hugging a man fully dressed as Santa, red coat, natural white beard and all. She looks completely happy, displaying her Elvis-like, diagonal grin, and so peaceful.

It's one of my favorite photos of her because it represents both her former and "new" self. Nana would never have hugged Santa, nor would she have seemed so at peace about the experience. It would be a forced, embarrassed smile. She normally avoided having her picture taken, and her pride, especially the desire to always seem "cool," often held her back from doing some fun things. This picture of her and Santa was the "new" Nana in living color. I liked this version, but it wasn't typical.

At the same time, it was the Nana we knew and loved. She hugged Santa because, to her core, she loved Christmas. It was by far her biggest holiday of the year. It took hours to open presents because she would buy a dozen or more for each of us. It was her greatest joy to give gifts, especially at Christmas, to decorate their home, to cook and prepare for our family to arrive on Christmas Day.

This photo reminds me that she was still Nana inside, no matter what changes happened.

I watched the 2014 movie, *Still Alice*, which won a Best Actress Oscar and Golden

Globe award.[17] It's the story of fictional character Alice Howland, a Harvard professor diagnosed with early onset Alzheimer's. This was the moment I truly came to understand the devastating effects of dementia, and it was a doozy.

As the title suggests, the entire point of the story was that no matter what she did, or said, how she behaved, or the point she no longer interacted at all . . . she was Still Alice, on the inside. Her life to that point, her experiences, family, and friends did not change.

What changed was her ability to communicate who she was, to display her personality.

I won't ruin the story for you—just read the book or watch the movie. But suffice it to say most of her circle could not deal with the effects of her illness, not even her husband. Change, especially when it's unexpected, makes people so uncomfortable they aren't sure how to react. There will always be some people who get it, who are perceptive enough to understand, and brave enough to carry on.

When that day comes for you, remember this—they are still the same person inside.

Summary Points

- The biggest loss for a dementia patient is not their memory, but their personality.

- Physical changes can present huge challenges, and they will need a lot of help.

- Watch for obsessive behaviors, but don't necessarily try to stop them—just help them to manage it. Distraction is a great strategy.

- Remember that underneath all the change, they are still the same person.

Having a solid mindset to understand that their physical, mental, and personality changes do not erase who they are inside will help prepare you both for the next step: transitioning them from a fully independent adult to a dependent person, someone who now relies on you for just about everything.

Chapter 6

Transition Time—Who, Me?

"Don't approach the problems that come along with dementia with dread. Instead, think positive, and find a solution."
- BOB DEMARCO

According to a 2020 report by the Alzheimer's Association,[18] nearly 6 million Americans live with the Alzheimer's form of dementia (AD). This includes 5.2 million people over 65, and 200,000 under age 65 who have younger-onset AD. One in eight people over 65 have AD.

The report also says 16 million Americans provide unpaid care for patients with Alzheimer's or other dementias—18.6 billion hours valued at $244 billion. What's the individual impact of investing all that time? There are many.

The article explains that caring for someone with dementia can damage your physical and psychological health. Negative health outcomes for family dementia caregivers, compared to non-caregiving people the same age, include higher rates of sleep disturbances and depression; poorer self-ratings of overall health status; and a 63% higher mortality rate.

It's unbelievably important that you make this transition into caregiving well.

I may not willingly jump onto this diagnosis bandwagon. You may have to pull me on, kicking and screaming. I won't want to believe or accept it, even if I have personal experience. I will make excuses and compensate to hide my symptoms. I might change my activities to limit our interactions . . . and hide my true condition.

Be patient with them. This is tough stuff, facing so much expected loss. In Chapter 1, I mentioned the 7-stage model of dementia, known as the Global Deterioration Scale/Reisberg Scale (GDS).[19] It describes the disease's impact in 7 stages, noting the memory and functional loss in each stage. By the time you have a diagnosis, they'll probably already be at stage 3-4, farther along than you might expect.

Helpful Strategies

There are several strategies I learned while caring for Nana, some through common sense, others through necessity, trial, and error. Everyone is different, and what works for some won't work for others. But these tactics helped me, and Nana, live and love well through her dementia. That's the main goal.

Liar, Liar: Most folks are taught to be honest. But remember, they won't be dealing with a full mental deck; they simply lack logic. Trying to reason with them will only lead to frustration for you both. Most people love stories, though, so making up stories, even lying at times, is often useful. If you figure out what catches and holds their interest, make up a story that can motivate them to do what's needed. This works, almost every time, if you've paid attention to your loved one and their disease progression. Mix in a bit of truth and their past, and you'll have even greater success.

Reminders Come in All Shapes and Sizes: Not to state the obvious, but they will forget a lot. And often what is forgotten, and when, won't make sense. It won't be intentional, so just expect it and be ready to help them. They may get angry at themself but lash out at you. Let me remind you—this is not intentional, so don't take it personally. Forgive them. I paid all of Nana's bills for her. One day she accused me of stealing her money. Talk about an ouch!

Nana watched TV for hours on end for most of my life, not just after her diagnosis. Since she worked full time at a mailing company, she would set her VCR every morning to record her favorite "soap operas" and court room show. She and that machine were best friends, and she could set it up in her sleep. That is, until dementia arrived.

I can't count how many arguments we had (what a waste of time, arguing with someone with dementia) about why, when, and how to record her shows. This was silly since she was retired, so there was no reason to record! One day, I found her sitting on the bed staring at the blank screen, angry. When I asked why, her reply was caustic. "I'm staring at this stupid TV because I can't get it to turn on and I figured eventually you might come in and help me!" She claimed to have been sitting there for two hours. I tried to remind her how to do it, then I tried to re-train her. I documented the instructions and put neon pink sticky notes on and around the TV to guide her. None of it mattered a hill of beans. She simply couldn't do it, and it drove her nuts. In her mind, we were both failing.

We had the same issue with her phone. We cut our land line, so I bought her and my dad a cell phone promoted by AARP. It was shiny red, with huge buttons, was wake-the-dead loud and quite simple. Or so I thought. I programmed it with names and numbers in large print. That much was appreciated. You know what the difficulty was, though? Recharging it. They never remembered to recharge it at night, and if they did, they'd forget to put it in their pocket the next morning. If it wasn't in their pocket, they couldn't hear it ring, no matter how loud I set the sound. The whole purpose of a cell was to avoid buying an emergency necklace (with the high monthly fee). If they kept a charged phone in their pocket, we could always communicate. That never worked like I hoped. Ever.

I recommend having multiple means of keeping me on task because as my dementia progresses, my need for help will increase. Plan to adapt. Calendar notes will change to colored stickers, then to one large daily page. Medication management will start by putting all the bottles together on my table, then move to your reminder calls. Then, you'll put the pills in a weekly pill box, by day, or next by am and pm by day. Pre-measured dosage packs or high-tech alarmed pill dispensers might be necessary. Eventually, someone will need to personally administer my meds.

You will give me lots of reminders. As I said, my needs will change often, increasing and sometimes decreasing. You'll remind me I need underwear, or that it goes under my pants, not on the outside. That I need to eat—I'll forget that a lot. Or that I already ate. That it's your birthday, or Mother's Day.

Some reminders won't work regardless of your efforts. My calendar may list a 9 a.m. visit with Dr. Jones tomorrow, and before bed we'll discuss the timing, you'll lay out my clothes, and I'll declare myself ready. But the next morning I won't wake up well, and I won't cooperate. I'll be cranky and slow, painfully slow, and we'll be late to the appointment. But if you're prepared for this, and have realistic expectations, you'll be more patient, which will help me become calmer, cooperative, and pleasant. A win-win for us both!

Avoid Frustration: I will repeat this a hundred times if necessary—frustration is your enemy, not the disease. During her acceptance phase, Nana's daily mantra was, "You think I'm crazy! I'm NOT crazy!" Since I seemed to be a slow learner through this, I tried to reason with her, even arguing at times. That was silly, but the truth. She was trying to keep her dignity, and I didn't see that. Her words hurt me, and I wanted her not to feel that way. I did wonder sometimes if I actually was treating her like she was crazy. It didn't matter because she sure believed it.

What's the remedy? Set realistic expectations and learn how to distract them. It can be so easy to distract a person with dementia. Nana's memory loss was sometimes a hidden blessing. If I told her I had to leave home for a while, and she became angry with me, it never lasted long. Five minutes later, she would forget about it. Shuffling out of her room, she would see me and declare what became our special exchange. "Sweetheart, you are the light of my life!" She'd smile and give me a hug with those loving, bony arms of hers. I learned if I could push through her negative reactions, it would be over soon. Frustration averted.

You can distract me in productive ways, other than just waiting for me to forget. I might like to do puzzles. Not complex ones, but surely any children's puzzle. I can work on them alone or as a partner project with you. Make a family picture puzzle for us to complete together . . . multiple times. Seriously, I won't mind at all because it will seem new every time.

Yes—as my disease progresses, experiences will always seem new. This can be fun for us. Driving down a "new" street or noticing a "new" store. I might see you wearing a "new" shirt, or say you served me a "new" recipe. And since everything seems new, I'll be excited about most things. Life will become a wonder for me. You can choose to be frustrated by this or amused. I highly recommend the latter. Enjoy showing me all these "new" things—I certainly will be enjoying them!

I digress though—squirrel. Here are a few activities that helped keep Nana occupied in a way she enjoyed, believe it or not. These will work with most folks. The result of the activity is not the goal; keeping their mind busy, doing something—anything—is.

- Folding our laundry. She loved to help others before her diagnosis, and interestingly, her joy in that never waned.
- Matching lost socks. At least she thought they matched, and I joyfully thanked her . . . and occasionally I even wore the mismatched pair she came up with.
- Sorting my box of extra buttons. By color, or by size, by number of holes. She enjoyed it all. You could also use LEGO blocks, a jar of extra screws, or nuts and bolts (make sure nothing sharp).
- Sorting the family pictures by person. Yes, this is a fruitless effort. She became distracted looking at each photo and would forget her goal. Plus, most photos include multiple people, so how could she sort by person? Regardless, she thoroughly enjoyed this.
- She kept every greeting card she ever received. Seriously. I must admit, I do this, too. Periodically, I would strategically leave them out for her to find. She would study each one as if it were new. Yes, sometimes she would cry. But usually for good, sentimental reasons.
- Go through photo albums with them. Tell them the stories of each picture. Try not to ask questions unless they share something relevant—they may not be able to answer, or understand, and might get frustrated.

Friends and Relatives: Among the most distressing effects of dementia is its impact on relationships. This is so clearly displayed in the movie I mentioned earlier, *Still Alice.* As your loved one's behavior changes, people around them won't know how to react or what to do. The most frequent question people asked me about Nana was, "Does she still know you?" Trust me when I say that is the last question you want to hear, but the first one on your own mind.

Helping me preserve relationships will require you to be patient and understanding of me and others. Prepare yourself mentally for the inevitable stares when we get to the restaurant, take my coat off, and my shirt is on inside out. Or the laughter when I say something totally inappropriate or out of character (which might be to curse), and everyone is laughing, or shocked, except me.

Teach those around us what to expect, how to react to me, and how best to support all of us. Teach them about dementia—that they don't have to fear the disease or me. Help them not to mourn my losses but to know me now, to laugh with me, to enjoy all the "new" experiences I'm having. To be kind to us.

Early on, I will enjoy going out, spending time with you, seeing and doing new things. But in time, we'll go out less because I'll be anxious, uncertain about what is happening, where we are, or what I'm supposed to do. This is normal, so don't be afraid. Just enjoy as much time together as possible while I can interact well.

Nana angrily accused me of being too embarrassed to be seen in public with her. That hurt me so much, especially since I was devoted to lovingly care for this woman who sacrificed so much for me. It's true that she almost always wore a soiled shirt and pants, so there might have been reason for embarrassment. Normally, she was spotless at home and in public. But her disease caused her to often spill, and she rarely even noticed. Often, I didn't notice until it was too late.

She wasn't trying to hurt me with her comments. She couldn't understand the impact, and her own survival instincts kicked in. Self-preservation, you know.

Again, since we've established I can be slow to learn, I tried to reason with her.

Don't do that. If it's a good day, try once and then move on. You don't win extra-

credit points for arguing. Pay close attention to their responses to know what to say, and when to stop.

This is especially important if you help them make a new friend—which, by the way, is a promising idea, though counterintuitive. When you do something new together, or visit a different place, watch them try to start up a conversation with a stranger. It will happen. And when it does, protect them; guide them with your comments and body language, join in, and ask carefully worded questions. Don't allow them to embarrass themself or unintentionally insult their new friend. Pay attention, and everything will be fine.

Above all, know that they love you, no matter what they might say or do. Things about your loved one will change. You can't stop that. They'll need so much of your help. You can't stop that, either. You know what else you can't stop, what will never change? At their core they're still the same.

Summary Points

- You both should start this journey with a positive perspective and keep it.

- Both of you will grieve at times as circumstances change. That's an okay place to visit, but you shouldn't live there.

- There are many strategies to help you both move forward. Don't be afraid to use them and create your own.

As if being a caregiver isn't already enough, there are many technical issues to work through. Legal decisions, paperwork, financial factors to consider—all of it complicated by the diagnosis. The earlier you take care of business—even years before their diagnosis—the better.

Chapter 7

The Technical, Legal Stuff

"You get better results if you plan long before there is a crisis."
- DAVID. J. FERRY, JR, ESQ.

Caring.com conducts annual surveys to determine how many folks have completed estate planning.[20] Traditionally, younger people are less likely to consider such topics. They may not realize they even have an estate. Researchers find that even 50-year-olds cannot envision their end of life. They may have basic life insurance, but for the majority, that's it.

In 2017, 60% of the over 55 demographic had a will in place. By 2020, that dropped to 48%. It's fascinating to see the most recent changes. Those who believe estate planning is especially important has dropped from 75% to 60%. Only a year earlier, just 1% of survey respondents said they had never thought about a will. In 2020, that number rose to 13%.

This is an abysmal trend, though not surprising. Few people spend time considering death or preparing for it . . . unless they are forced. Thanks to your loved one's diagnosis, you both will be forced.

Here's the Good News and the Bad News

First, the bad news. After Nana's diagnosis, her gerontologist's support staff looked me in the eye and asked this, "Does your mom have her estate documents in order? A will, living will, trust, power of attorney, those types of arrangements?"

My parents' will granted guardianship for me to Uncle Glen and Aunt Joyce. In other words, it was an out-of-date document, considering I was 52 years old at the time of Nana's diagnosis. "No," I replied, "She does not. Basically, everything goes to me, and I'll be providing their care."

My response must have been unusual, because she seemed confused. "So, you don't have any siblings, or anyone who might fight you over their estate ownership?"

"Nope, I don't think so." I'm an only child, so this was an easy conversation.

She then popped the bad news: once diagnosed with dementia, Nana could not legally sign or commit to anything. Technically, it was now too late for her to sign the recommended legal documents.

The good news was we were early in this process, and given my status as the only child and full heir (after my dad, of course), I would be able to get documents executed quickly.

I may not be too happy about being declared legally unfit. Be sure we start this journey while I still have enough reason to understand why I need to hand you the reins. Life will be much easier if we are proactive rather than reactive.

Even though you might have legal and medical authority over my life, please don't wield that power like a sledgehammer. There is no need to flaunt it, to rub it in my face, or to overrule me at every turn. Remember, one of our goals throughout this experience is respect. As your mother, I've earned it. As followers of Christ, you're called to honor me—it's one of the Big Ten, you know.

How do you show respect, practically speaking? Let them think they are making the decision, even if they're not. Ask their opinion, point out pros and cons. They may surprise you and choose wisely. And if not, it's not much different than dealing with a teenager, or a toddler—discuss options, but in the end, you choose. Just because they make a choice, you don't have to follow it. They won't remember.

Eeney, Meeny, Miny, Moe

You'll have many decisions to make for your loved one in this stage. One of the first is who is in charge. There are right and wrong ways to do this.

Suppose you have sibling caregivers. The wrong approach is to reach no agreement at all, for one to get mad and take over, and for the rest to exit in a huff while complaining about the "power broker" in the room.

The right approach, in my experience, is for one person to be the legal representative. They can then delegate the monitoring, medical, and social responsibilities in a fair way. Adjustments can be made as needed depending on the disease progression and needs. But this is a good starting point. It's not helpful for one caregiver to feel more burdened than another, or at least not more than might be natural. Consider taking turns on various areas, involving other family or friends as they are willing. Hopefully, your loved one will be a sweet, not unruly, patient.

The Keys to the Kingdom: The All About Me Folder

Before any diagnosis or crisis, make sure you have a paper or digital folder where you can access their important documents. (In fact, you should have the same set up yourself). It should include insurance information (homeowners, cars, life, medical, etc.), their medical history, asset ownership titles, birth certificate for them and their spouse, their marriage license, and the death certificate of any predeceased spouse. These documents may be needed to manage and settle the estate or to claim the life insurance.

As for their assets, generally it's best to put everything—house, car, personal belongings, cash, and investment accounts—in a family trust. Do this well before any dementia diagnosis. But if that was not done, you can work with an attorney to set up a trust and assign bank account access so you can pay their bills. Without cash access, it will be difficult to help manage their finances.

The Keys to the Kingdom: The Experts

A lawyer joke (courtesy of jokes4us.com):

Q: What do you get when you cross a librarian with a lawyer?

A: All the information you need, but you can't understand a word of it.

An accountant joke (courtesy of jokes4us.com):

Q: What is the definition of "accountant"?

A: Someone who solves a problem you didn't know you had in a way you don't understand.

Why the humor break? Because I want to soften you up for this piece of advice: even though you may not think so, you would benefit by consulting with an elder law attorney and a financial advisor. And it won't be cheap. Remember our earlier discussion about our village, the support community we need to build? You'll need these experts.

My husband and I are both CPAs. We know tax and estate law can change with every political administration. There's no good reason to pay a penny more in inheritance tax than necessary. All jokes aside, they truly can help. You'll find great folks you trust who can offer sound guidance.

Whether they have an estate worth $10 or $10,000 (I know—setting the bar a little low), there are strategies that will reduce any tax burden. Factors like capital gains, gifting assets to family (amount and timing), who is titled as owner—these types of considerations should be addressed. Ideally, before your loved one is diagnosed. Don't be afraid to bring it up. If they accuse you of being a gold digger and after their money, don't be offended. That's a sign you should act quickly on the legal matters and then get them evaluated.

My will should name someone as executor. The estate executor manages all the steps to finalize my estate, such as paying last bills, notifying proper parties, distributing assets, and a bit more. Hopefully, I have chosen someone before my health goes south. Initially, it would be my spouse. But I should name a secondary if they are unable to serve as executor. It could be you, or another family member, but that's not required. We should discuss this early so key players know the plans. This is not a popularity contest. I should choose the person most capable, available, and willing to do this. You as executor would cost much less than naming an attorney, so keep that in mind if your goal is preserving assets. Who knows—maybe we'll have a friend who could capably serve on a pro bono basis.

The Keys to the Kingdom: Funeral Arrangements

Millennials (those born between 1980-1994) are a "death positive generation" according to a 2020 article written by Eleanor Cummins and published on Vox.com.[21] What is that, you say? Apparently, millennials are doing their funeral planning now to rescue their loved ones from the financial and emotional burden of having to do that later.

Not surprising since millennials value social issues over institutions and believe in activism and change. It's fascinating to explore the innovative ways millennials are driving change in the death business.

I am a Boomer. As a group, my generation stubbornly delayed any funeral planning well into our 60's through 70's, at best. Usually we waited until someone close died and we were forced. The funeral staff offered us a discounted "two-for-one," which we bought in the midst of our grief and distraction. But hey, at least we had some of it planned, right?

Nana refused to discuss anything related to death. I got her to do it by saying my husband and I were writing a new will and making funeral plans and needed her opinions. I uncovered all the information I needed without her realizing it.

In our circle, there was one "go to" funeral home. Most people we knew used it, including my dad for his sister and mother. When my dad passed, we called that facility to retrieve his body from the hospital. I confess—I didn't give this any thought. We received the call that he was crashing, rushed to the hospital, and he was already gone. The nurse said two things to me: I am so sorry, and who should we call to pick up his body?

At the time, I wasn't prepared to make that decision, and you may not be, either. The nurse was waiting for an answer, so I said the first thing that came to mind—call the old standby funeral home. No research, no knowledge of new providers, no concept of cost. Nana was already diagnosed and unable to make these decisions. It was up to me.

This was a lousy approach. The whole experience was horrible for me and for Nana. My dad's funeral was twice the cost of Nana's, the staff was less compassionate and patient, and they were totally unwilling to adjust for even our most reasonable requests. My experience planning Nana's service was far better, actually pleasant.

There are multiple decisions involved in end-of-life planning, and likely your loved one will have opinions about it all. Ask their wishes early, while they're still able to remember and have some amount of logic. The top issues to discuss include:

- Burial, or cremation, or both
- In ground or mausoleum
- Open or closed casket (which can happen with both physical burial and cremation)
- Public or family service
- Who speaks, and if you will have clergy participate
- What is the service like—speaking, slide show, music? For both my parents' funerals, I made a music CD to play during the visitation, and before the service, of all their favorite songs. It was so eclectic and served two purposes— to share a bit about them with visitors and to comfort me. My dad's was mostly 1940s big band and ballads. Nana's was hymns, gospel music, and Elvis. Hearing their music comforted me then and now.
- Obituary, service brochure and thank you notes, guest book (they have packages for everything)
- What happens to their remains if cremated?

I was fortunate to have a list of funeral songs Nana had written down after my dad died. The cemetery sold us a double plot at that time, so we had burial covered. But we made mistakes. As a veteran, my dad could have been buried in any national cemetery for free, with the choice of buying the adjacent plot for Nana at a low cost. We have a national cemetery in our city. Because we had little time, and did not preplan, we paid thousands for a plot we could have received for free. I did learn in time that, as a veteran, his headstone would be provided free by the U.S. Government. That alone saved Nana a bundle.

There are practical and financial reasons to plan the funeral in this early stage. I must make a plug for Newcomer Funeral Homes, who we used for Nana's arrangements. A friend mentioned her husband was a mortician (I had no idea) and worked for Newcomer. So, when Nana passed and the nurse asked me who to call, I knew how to respond. I trusted my friend and called her husband. Newcomer was wonderful, reasonably priced, extremely caring, wonderful (did I already say that?) —I could not have asked for a better experience, odd as that may sound. They are on my funeral "to do" list—you must call Newcomer. They have locations around the USA.

Summary Points

- Plan early and get expert help (the neighbor or friend can support you, but not direct you).

- Don't fight about who legally takes which caregiving role. Do what's best for all.

- There are a few "Keys to the Kingdom" that will guide future decisions—the "all about me" folder, deciding who does what, and funeral arrangements.

So far, we've started the medical planning, begun transitioning to this new reality, and handled the business aspects of your loved one's life. You still have one more area to address—the practical, day-to-day management of their care. Paying for this, managing medical care, and watching their ability to live on their own. I realize it's a lot, this technical, legal stuff. But you can do this together, early. Life will be simpler as you face the practicalities of day-to-day care.

Chapter 8

Getting Down to Business:
The Practical Stuff

*"The disease might hide the person underneath, but there's still a person
in there who needs your love and attention."*
- JAMIE CALANDRIELLE

In the last chapter, I mentioned you should divide and conquer the
various aspects of your loved one's care. This should be a fair
delegation. But like with parenting, fair does not necessarily mean
equal. When that time comes, each person helping you may be at
different stages in their life. Be considerate of that reality as you work
together.

Count the Cost

*Getting old is not cheap. Disease and dying are part of the money-making
machine called health care. I should have saved, invested in long-term
care insurance, compiled enough resources to cover my expenses ... in
combination with Social Security, which I pray daily still exists. I repeat:
I should have saved. Don't assume I did.*

According to Genworth's Cost of Care projections for Indiana,
by 2040 when I turn age eighty, the monthly average cost for an in-

home health aide will be nearly $8,100. Each month. Adult Day Care will run $3,700, assisted living $7,400, a nursing home semi-private room $12,100. A private room is estimated at $13,700 per month. Costs tend to rise about 3% per year.[22]

That's why families should plan well in advance and use estate planning. Why you should plan now rather than later. Failing to plan could mean there are inadequate resources to provide proper care, and certainly nothing to leave to descendants.

This becomes another area we must discuss now, particularly since circumstances change over time. Bill, a friend's father, saved faithfully during his life. When dementia hit, his family had nearly all options on the table. They were able to choose a wonderful memory care facility for his final days. Jane, another friend's mom, and her family had limited resources … and thus limited options. In the end, her family and friends took turns providing in-home care with a few hours of paid nursing staff. They were exhausted, frustrated, and unable to enjoy her final days in any way.

When Nana and my dad were sixty, I encouraged them to buy long-term care insurance. We had a quote for $120 per month for an indexed policy—one that had adequate coverage to pay nursing costs then and would increase over time at a rate indexed to, or equal to, long-term care inflation.

Unfortunately, their health, while not awful, did result in a denied application. They refused to pursue it further. They had no assets at the end, having sold their home and contributed most of the proceeds toward construction of our joint, family residence. The rest they mismanaged. When Nana needed day care, my family secretly paid part of it because she would have been mortified to know we were having to help. When she broke her hip and needed nursing home care to rehab, she had no resources other than social security. When my dad died, his already small pension was reduced to the spousal rate of less than $300 per month. We had no choice but to explore Medicaid and other government funded options to pay for her care.

If your loved one doesn't have adequate resources or insurance to pay for needed care, you should make a plan.

One side note: You might consider long-term care plans for yourself, too. It is not just older folks who use long-term care. According to a 2010 article published by NPR, between 2000–2010, the fastest growing population in nursing homes were those aged 31–64, rising to 14.2% of all residents nationwide.[23] Accidents resulting in disability or experiencing severe illness and disease can leave you unable to live on your own for some period of time, or for the remainder of your days. It could wipe out everything you own and leave your family in financial ruin without planning. Not to sound like an insurance ad, but coverage is so inexpensive (comparatively) when you are young, and setting aside savings or investing for long-term is so simple to do. It's at least worth a conversation with a financial planner.

Doctor Management

True story: I was at my annual gynecology exam and mentioned that I experienced sharp chest pains when laying on my left side. My doc, with decades of experience not only in his field, but with me, offered this wise counsel, "Then, don't lay on your left side."

My point is that I asked a gynecologist a cardiology question. Yes, they do all go to medical school. But at some point, their specialties overtake general knowledge. I should have known better. Then again, he did ask me if I had any concerns. Those pains were a concern.

As you move through the disease stages, an increasing number of specialists will enter the picture. In case you think managing the doctors is simply a matter of finding a good calendar app, hear me out.

In Chapter 2, I shared how Nana ended up with an endocrinologist for her osteoporosis and an ENT for her thyroid. There were many other examples of this as we all worked to find and connect her medical dots, so to speak.

When I took over her medical care, she had three physicians: her primary, heart, and kidney doctors. Her nephrologist (kidney doctor) was an older, interesting man. He spent as much time as it took each visit for Nana to spend her words; he was truly kind and patient, extremely observant, and always watching. He listened to what she said, certainly, but more importantly he asked questions that allowed him to see how she answered, her body language, and he used those clues to help guide her care. I loved that guy.

Through her regular bloodwork and his probing questions, he suspected she had vascular issues brewing in her left leg. So, off we went to a vascular doctor. Turned out her main vein was literally broken in that leg ... missing a section likely due to years of pre-OSHA standing on concrete. She had insufficient blood flow down her left leg into her foot.

Understand, Nana complained about back and leg pain for most of my life. Post-diagnosis, it was challenging to know which complaints to take seriously. These pains were usually attributed to spinal issues, and in fact, one of her quarterly visits was to a spine doctor who administered pain management steroid shots. His specialty was a doozy—Anesthesiology specializing in Minimally Invasive Spinal Diagnostics and Therapeutics.

Because of her history, I paid little attention to her leg pain complaints. She had pain pills, and we were in between steroid shots, so some level of discomfort was expected. But the news that her circulation was, well, missing, was a game changer on several levels.

In addition to regular monitoring visits, he sent us to a podiatrist to cut her toenails. The poor circulation had left them extremely thick and impossible to cut, which caused ingrown nails and more pain. Another monthly doctor visit.

The vascular doc recommended she have a leg stent inserted to restore blood flow. By this time, she was developing leg and foot sores, and the toes were turning dark. But she needed her thyroid surgery, too, so we delayed the leg stent so she could recover from the thyroid surgery.

Eventually, she had a second leg stent surgery, a heart catheterization procedure because her pre-op tests showed a heart anomaly, and shortly before her death, an amputation (enter another doctor—orthotic). The physician list multiplied.

A Curse or a Blessing?

Each different physician means a minimum of six visits, with some requiring monthly follow-ups. By the time of her passing, Nana's doctor list included 17 different physicians, not including the rehab hospital primary doctor. So, a total of 18, I guess. That is a ton of medical appointments to manage.

The bad news is these take a fair amount of time. I will probably be slow to get ready (it takes me an average of one hour to "get ready" for any outing), and slow to transport. Doctors rarely run on time, although I must say my specialists did a pretty good job. Except for the kidney doc, but I didn't mind since he was so intentional about talking with me.

The good news is this gives us some wonderful, special time together. Since you won't be able to rush the process, plan to use these events to talk with me. Share your own news, ask me questions about whatever I might remember, discuss current events (I have always been a depository of cultural news, so I'll love to discuss events, entertainment, sports).

I suggest you schedule no more than two appointments each week, preferably in the morning. They'll have greater clarity then. Afterward, take them out to eat, or stop by a store to pick up something, anything. It will be good for them to see other people, to experience normal life. And time with you will be a lifeline for them, the main thread to connect their past with their present. Time is short and precious. All these appointments? They are a gift.

I should point out a big, potential road hazard—just because the doctors are experts in their fields doesn't mean they are experts in ALL fields. I started this chapter with a joke about this.

While I certainly was concerned about Nana's declining cognitive level, my first motivation to involve a gerontologist was care coordination. I wanted one doctor who could track everyone to make sure they didn't work against Nana's best interests, unintentionally. Really—they don't know what they don't know, right? Asking her was a waste of breath—even in her pre-dementia days she had trouble explaining what all the doctors were doing for her, or even remembering all of them. I had to show her the x-rays to prove to her she had a shoulder replaced. She had no recollection at all, and replied, "Well, no wonder my shoulder hurts sometimes!" In her dementia, she rolled with the punches.

Nana's PCP eventually took over the coordination of all her doctors by receiving and reading all case notes. She regularly informed me about any potential care conflicts, and all Nana's doctors received communication from the PCP's office. It's so important to have one doctor who can oversee everything that may be ongoing in their medical care. It was common for her many doctors to mention each other's treatment regimens during our appointments. This helped me know the strategy was working.

In many ways, caring for Nana was easier for me because I had no siblings. Yes, as an only child with no other family around, my husband and I had to do everything. E-V-E-R-Y-T-H-I-N-G. If you have siblings or very close relatives, you could spread the load.

At the same time, I was able to make plans without having to consider other people's schedules (coordination with our family calendar is a given). You and others you involve must work together to manage the medical calendar. Even if your loved one has a spouse available, they'll need help. It might be too much for them to manage alone at the age they may be. I am confident you'll figure out the best way to do this, and I have resources listed in a planned companion workbook to help. The key takeaway is to be considerate and humble in working with others. Remember—fair is not equal.

Watch Like a Hawk

A doctor joke, courtesy of onelinefun.com: "When I told the doctor about my loss of memory, he made me pay in advance."

I can't stress enough how important it is to keep a sense of humor when you are caring for a dementia patient. The disease offers an opportunity to see life from a new and unique perspective. Take advantage of this.

In Chapter 3, I shared a behavior log template to help you keep track of your loved one's behavior. It's simple, but effective. Remember what they say about data: GIGO (garbage in, garbage out). A behavior log will only be helpful if the information noted is complete, accurate, and timely.

You need a way(s) to gather this information. There are many technology tools available to record data through text or by voice, and certainly there are health apps you can use. Just remember to record what you see and hear. Try to arrange for someone to contact them every day. A mix of voice, personal, and video contact would be ideal. It's always good to see others faces and expressions. But voice can also be very insightful as it removes visual distractions.

What should you track, and which metrics should you use? Here are a few suggestions.

- How long does it take them to complete routine tasks and complex tasks?
- Do they respond to calls quickly, and is their response time slowing down?
- Are their dependable traits changing (such as personal cleanliness, ability to recognize when something is dirty), or do they no longer care?
- Are they having balance issues, tripping, needing a cane or walker?
- Is their manner of speech changing, cadence slowing, having greater difficulty tracking in conversation?
- Are they safe performing normal living activities at home (cooking, cleaning, stairs, or dressing and showering)?

Most of these observations are subjective, and everyone may not agree on what they see. I understand. It'll be very hard to see my abilities fail. Remember what I said about a sense of humor. I have never been afraid to laugh at myself, and I hope this doesn't change in my dementia. But regardless of my attitude, be intentional to see and point out the humor in our experiences whenever possible.

There is no room for shame in our care community. Funny story: As I mentioned earlier, Nana was extremely proud and independent. She needed no one. This aspect of her personality took a 180 degree turn in her dementia, and that was a huge blessing to me. Nana's left leg was amputated because we couldn't permanently restore the circulation and stop the intruding gangrene—we had to save her life.

My mother, who would not even let you open the door for her and would have been mortified at the thought of losing a limb, never once complained about her amputation. In fact, she asked us several times to remove it to stop her growing pain.

On her second day post-op, her nurse checked the stump and redressed it as she did every few hours. Nana was a trooper through it all, very cooperative and pleasant. When the sheet was pulled back, Nana was surprised and declared, "Oh, look, they cut off my leg!" and started to laugh. Maybe this was one of those "you had to be there moments" but trust me—this was hilarious at the time! Pre-dementia, she would have been mean, angry, and at best, difficult to manage with such an invasive and complete loss of independence, from her perspective anyway.

But the look on her face, the surprise in her voice at the realization (remember, everything can be new to a dementia patient) of this missing appendage was downright funny. We all laughed, and it became one of my favorite memories, odd as that sounds. Even though I was pained because of what we had to do, she reminded us all that it was just a leg, as she said, and we needed to keep that perspective.

Laughter is always one of the best medicines. It's not just a cliché.

Summary Points

- Start planning now for the cost of their care, how you will pay for it and who will pay (yes, this is a real question).

- Have a system to manage their medical appointments, and aim to turn those into adventures, not inconveniences.

- You need a tool to track their behavior closely—it will guide the doctors and care.

At this point, it should be crystal clear how dementia is affecting them. I expect it will be affecting you, too, as their caregiver. As you enter the next stage of their disease, let's discuss the roller coaster you'll experience—changes for them, decisions to be made for both your benefit, and how to protect you along the way.

Part II

---⊗---

The Middle Stage

Chapter 9

Caregiving: There's a Right Way and a Wrong Way

"Courage is not living without fear. Courage is being scared to death and doing the right thing anyway."
- ARGO, 2012

Movies and television speak to me. They always have and probably always will. I especially love those that are self-revealing—surprises that I wasn't looking for and maybe didn't even want to find. Surprises that unveil those "aha" moments bringing joy, relief, and sometimes pain.

NBC's dramedy, *Zoey's Extraordinary Playlist,* surprised me.[24] Often. It's an intriguing exploration of interpersonal and family dynamics, told through the impact of terminal illness and the songs that sometimes play in our heads. This is a very, very simplistic summary. But it will suffice to set the stage.

In the episode titled "Zoey's Extraordinary Silence," the lead character, Zoey, had conversations with her dying father's in-home caregiver, Howie, about her dad's health. Dad was failing quickly, and Zoey dreaded his inevitable passing. Howie was a professional specializing in end-of-life situations. He'd been in this situation many times before, and Zoey wanted to know how she should manage the situation.

Howie's Pearls of Wisdom

Successfully dealing with terminal diseases like dementia requires a certain perspective. Watching your loved one failing will often be agonizing. What was Howie's advice to Zoey? That the caregiving experience teaches you how incredibly special every day is—to realize it's a blessing to breathe on our own, to get up and walk. To talk, or not. Our choice. Every day.

At the same time, everyone is created so uniquely. There's no recipe for care, and it can be maddening to know the right way, and the wrong way, to be a caregiver.

Knowing the difference will be vital to successfully navigating, and growing, through this journey.

Early on I'll lose my ability to self-advocate. Some days, you'll desperately want to do things for me because I'm slow, clunky, and you're in a hurry or are afraid for me. But I must keep trying on my own. Remember that. I must push myself to do uncomfortable and new things to have the best chance of holding my disease at bay as long as possible. Other times, I may want you to do something, maybe everything, for me because I am afraid, or slow, embarrassed, not feeling well —there may be a million reasons why. And you won't feel like helping me. Deep down, I understand. It's alright.

I am ashamed to admit this, but there were times I hid from Nana. I could hear her slippers shuffling through the bathroom and into the kitchen. When I was especially tired and emotionally raw, I would slip into the laundry room, confident when she didn't see me in the kitchen, she would shuffle back into her bedroom. I simply had nothing to offer and couldn't bear to snap at her, even though I knew she would forget all about it in five minutes. But she would remember the feelings, and I would remember I hid.

That is the wrong way to care for your loved one.

Yes, this reaction might be understandable. But it's not excusable. Instead of feeling shame for the mistakes you make, I want to help you grow through this journey. I want to help you have joy through knowing the right ways to provide care. We'll spend a lot of time in these chapters talking about the right ways, because it will be lifegiving.

Noah and Ally

Another movie example (spoiler alert), *The Notebook*, by Nicholas Sparks, is thought to be a prime example of the American tearjerker love story.[25] Noah meets Ally, falls hard for Ally, loses Ally, gets Ally, and they live a long, incredibly happy life together—until Alzheimer's enters the picture, wreaking havoc.

In the story, their relationship illustrates love in a multitude of ways, but none so moving as the moment you realize the older man and woman dancing together, holding each other so tenderly, are Noah and Ally. Noah's compassion is clear when you realize how much he's has sacrificed to care for Ally, solely to experience those fleeting moments of her twinkly eyes and loving recognition; the sacrifices he made so he could comfort her when she is mentally absent, afraid, and sees Noah as a stranger.

I believe this is the right way to provide care. With humility, patience, an awareness of living, and the courage to sacrifice, to make tough choices. And to laugh.

I searched for "dementia care" books on Amazon, pulling up over 4,000 results. On Google, dementia had over 81 million hits. There is no shortage of information about the disease, and probably every aspect of it—so many books saying *what* to do in dementia care. Few are telling us *how* to do it. There is a significant difference.

What to Do vs. How to Do It

Here's an analogy to explain what I mean. If you bake muffins, your recipe will say to mix flour, sugar, eggs, milk, maybe nuts or berries. You mix ingredients, pour into a muffin tin, and bake. Sounds simple enough. That's all you need to make muffins—the ingredients.

Experienced bakers know this isn't enough. You need those items, but mixing alone won't create a great muffin. The "how" needed for the muffins to be light, airy, and delightful includes separating the wet and dry ingredients. The "how" requires you to make a hollow in the center of your dry ingredients, slowly pour the wet ingredients into the hollow, and to mix ever so gently, not beating it, until it is almost mixed, but not completely.

That's the difference between *what to do* and *how to do*, lifting our efforts from ordinary into extraordinary through our attitude, planning, and imagination. Knowing *how* to give care will help carry you through both the simple, and the dramatic, changes that are coming.

Lori La Bey, CSA, is the founder, president, and CEO of Alzheimer's Speaks, a Minneapolis-based advocacy group that provides education and support for those dealing with Alzheimer's disease and dementia.[26] After 30 years living with and caring for her mother through dementia, Lori developed a tool she calls Your Memory Chip ™ that provides guidance to know what to focus on in caregiving and why.[27]

Following Lori's guidelines, ask yourself these questions before any interaction with your loved one, especially if there's a chance their behavior, responses, or attitude might be challenging, irritating, or possibly driving you to anger.

- What do you want them to know? *Really* want them to know. Is information the most important thing, or what they make you feel like? Or is it more important that they feel loved, that you love them no matter what? Remember— they will remember how they feel even if they don't remember why.

- What should you focus on? Clue: It isn't getting somewhere on time, how they inconvenience you, or if they look embarrassingly silly. Lori wisely points out the Big Three questions that should be your focus.

  o Is Mom/Dad safe?

  o Is Mom/Dad happy?

  o Is Mom/Dad pain-free?

- What memories do you want to hold? Their laugh, sense of humor, silliness? How much they love musicals, *Die Hard* movies and Marvel action heroes, and all things Disney?

Try as you may, you won't be able to stop them from repeating themself. No amount of effort will correct their misperceptions. Expecting them to understand, to change, to cooperate will generally lead to pain for you both. So instead of wasting your energies and emotions trying, ask Lori's Your Memory Chip™ questions. It will help keep you on the road to sweet memories and leave regrets in the dump heap where they belong.

Summary Points

- There is a right and wrong way to care for your loved one—it's a balancing act between their dependence on self and their dependence on you.

- Doing this right requires humility, patience, an awareness of life, courage to sacrifice, and the ability to laugh, to help them see the humor in each day.

- Tools like Your Memory Chip™ can guide your interactions and reduce frustration.[28] For every interaction, ask how it affects their safety, happiness, and pain level.

It's so important to understand me and what I need. To understand what will help, and what won't, for me to live well through my disease. Our challenge is change—constant and erratic change. It seems the minute you figure me out, I'll be different.

Chapter 10

The Fork(s) in the Road(s)

"If you come to a fork in the road, take it."
- YOGI BERRA

Occasionally, I wander down the baby product aisles at Target. There's an overwhelming array of styles and brands of wipes and pacifiers. I think my parents had maybe two options for anything.

When I was in junior high, my dad had a part-time job restocking area grocery stores with Gerber baby food. Each summer, I helped him find Gerber cases on the delivery dock, move them to the store sales floor, and restock the shelves. There were so many types of veggies, fruits, meats. Too many apparently, because we frequently threw out expired jars.

The changes in infant care guidance over the course of my baby-rearing years often left my head spinning. My older two boys slept on their tummies—doctor's orders. Eight years later, we were told our youngest son had to sleep on his side to be safe. Use a pacifier, don't use a pacifier. Potty train by age two. Forget that—use a pull-up (diaper companies' huge conspiracy to sell us diapers forever). Theories on feeding, education, discipline—it all changed in a mere eight years.

Change Is the Name of the Game

I researched synonyms for the word "change." According to dictionary.com, they include: development, advance, adjustment, diversity, shift, transition, variation, switch, revolution, reversal, innovation, modification, difference, transformation, revision, turnaround, evolve, reduce, resolve, reform.

There are probably as many variations of the word change as there are changes you'll experience during your loved one's illness. There will be many changes, and they'll affect you both. I've mentioned a few already. But let's dive into some of the less obvious and perhaps more interesting, in no particular order.

Driving

They'll have to stop driving . . . earlier than they think they should. In Chapter 3, I shared about taking Nana's keys away. Let's hope you have a much easier time of it. But make no mistake, this must be done, for their safety and others, and to protect us legally.

Credit Cards

You'll need to take these from me, or I may spend every penny I don't have. One excellent choice —leave me with one card that has a tiny limit or has been cancelled. Every time I try to use it and it's declined, I'll complain about the company but quickly forget. Allowing me to have an active card, in my possession, with a higher limit, is like letting a toddler play with a sharp knife. You are not just asking for trouble; you are guaranteeing it.

Doctor Talk

There will be this awkward phase where they are conversant and seem coherent. The doctor and staff will direct questions to them, not to you. Some of this is out of respect, which is all well and good. The problem is, your loved one won't be completely objective or terribly truthful. They won't truly recall what they've done or haven't done, how they feel or what they said. If you don't fill in the gaps when needed, their medical care will suffer. Sometimes at Nana's appointments the staff completely ignored me. I was offended, but you don't need to be. Anticipate it, and patiently insert yourself into the conversation. Eventually, Nana refused to respond, and, gesturing to me, would say, "Talk to her—she knows better than me."

Physical Therapy

If one of my doctors does not order physical therapy, then, please, plan to do regular physical activity with me on your own. Walking on your arm, chair leg lifts and stretches, lifting small hand weights. There are free workouts online specifically for seasoned citizens. I need those endorphins running amok to help me stay positive and as physically strong as possible.

Physical Surroundings

You may be familiar with baby and toddler home safety gear, like electrical outlet plugs, furniture corners, stair gates, and such. The details may be a bit different, but it's the same concept—as their cognitive ability declines, along with their mobility, they will be less safe everywhere. Routinely examine places and rooms they frequent to look for dangers.

If I lose my balance, is there always something nearby to grab for steadiness? Are there rugs or furniture that could trip me? Are things I need close and easily accessible, so I don't have to reach or climb? Is my phone always available, or maybe a safety pendant, watch, or other connected device that can alert others I need help? Some steps you take may be basic, common sense to you, but they won't be to me. I will always think of myself as age 30 or 40, grab a chair, and get on it to reach that bowl on the top shelf. My reality and my memory will be at odds, so I'll need you to fill that gap.

Assistance Devices

Monitor the need for assistive devices like a cane, walker, scooter, tub/shower handrails, a potty chair, or bedside toilet (with arms) that can serve multiple purposes. There are so many adaptive items that can help them be safe and manage whatever challenges they will have. Be observant. And if what they need isn't available, improvise or invent it! There is always a way. Always. A word of warning, though. They may not be eager to use some of these items, so your creativity will be important. If they don't like the walker, let's spruce it up with awesome duct tape, bike streamers, or a bell. Whatever—just as long as it's colorful and fun. Nana loved such frills.

Laundry Multiplies

Because of spills and incontinence, you will have much more laundry to wash, so plan how you will manage that. One solution is to buy them more clothes so they don't need washing as often. (Now that's what I like to hear!) They will spill more when eating, or while doing pretty much anything. And they won't notice that very well. Be watching for ways to help them stay clean and presentable.

Getting Dressed

Another area that will decline is their ability to dress themself. One of my favorite poems is titled, "Warning" by Jenny Joseph.[29] It starts like this:

> *When I am an old woman I shall wear purple*
> *With a red hat which doesn't go, and doesn't suit me.*
> *And I shall spend my pension on brandy and summer gloves*
> *And satin sandals, and say we've no money for butter.*

I love this poem. Bold, brazen, honest. Plus, I love purple. As for clothing, at first, they'll be fine, or at least what you typically expect from them. Then they'll begin to mismatch clothing—colors, styles, that kind of thing. They may put on a heavy sweater with shorts. Or try to wear a winter coat on an 80° day. This might be due to confusion, oversight, or simply not giving a hoot. They may start forgetting items, like socks or underwear.

In the second year after her diagnosis, I began to lay Nana's clothes out for her each night because she was painfully slow in the morning as she decided what to wear, and she would forget to put on clean undies . . . or wear two pairs. So, we would select tomorrow's outfit together each evening. I would make it fun by picking things that I knew she would think odd, or I would make fun of myself in some way. Anything to help her laugh. But my ulterior motives were to preserve her respect and get her moving along a bit faster the next day.

Toilet Trouble

This contributes to the laundry issues. Think of all the decisions you make, automatically, to drive a car. Over time it becomes instinct, without conscious effort, for the most part. Toileting is similar. But eventually, they will lose track of the order of steps, or what needs to be done.

Think about this process for a minute. You feel the urge, find the room, turn on the light, shut the door, take down your pants, open the lid, sit, use the toilet paper to wipe, remember that you should clean up, know how to wipe and do it thoroughly, put the soiled paper in the toilet, stand up and put your pants back on, flush, wash your hands, open the door, turn off the light and leave.

There are multiple opportunities to mess this up, and they'll need help—less early on, but you should keep an eye out. Will that be uncomfortable? Yes. At some point either you get over it, your spouse or others will help, or you'll hire an aide. Bathing falls into this category, too. Their skin may become very thin and dry. Help them to be clean, moisturized, and healthy.

Instructions

They'll forget how to do the common and complex, how to find items that are near and dear to them, or their purpose if they do find them. In the movie adaptation of *Still Alice*,[30] Alice senses that she is forgetting especially important matters. So, she decides to record a video of herself explaining what to do, then she can refer to that when she forgets. Best laid plans, though. When the time comes, she forgets how to use the computer.

I'll need instructions, more often over time. I realize this is like a broken record, but you must watch me carefully and understand what you see. If you rush our time together, you may miss important things.

Pills, Pills . . . Pills

I'll probably take several medications. Maybe we'll get lucky and science will develop a personalized prescription cocktail that combines all my medications for a given time into one pill or liquid dose. Or better yet, a fruit flavored gummy! But if not, I'll need help to manage meds.

In Chapter 6, I mentioned how needs progress in this area. Practically speaking, a daily pill box works well. There are many types of these, some with one little box per day for a week, others with three to four boxes per day and three weeks. I used this big mama for Nana. It took several hours to fill the boxes, plus a fair amount of concentration not to mix it up. At the prescribed time, I would bring her water and remind her it was time.

Initially, I would leave her then. Eventually, I realized that if I left, she would get distracted and forget to take the pills. So, we sat together until all the pills were taken. That irritated her to no end, and she complained that I was treating her like a baby, not trusting her, that kind of thing. But it had to be done. Those medications kept her going for years.

Sleeping, or Not

As people age, they tend to sleep less. But in truth, according to sleepeducation.org, seniors need seven to nine hours a night, much like younger adults.[31] The problem is, they don't produce enough melatonin, the sleep hormone, so they have trouble getting and staying asleep. There are other contributing factors, like aches and pains, having to go potty more often, and being unable to fall back to sleep. Natural hearing loss helps; sounds don't bother them as much.

But a big issue in this area is what happens while they sleep—the nightmares—and the hallucinations when they're awake. These are real and frightening. I can't stress enough that you should do research to prepare . . . and expect that you may still be caught off-guard when they happen.

For some patients, these delusions worsen in their disease's later stages. Nana's nightmares were terrifying, and it was difficult to calm her. Fortunately, this phased out over time and with a slight medication adjustment.

On occasion, Nana's delusions were conversations with friends or family that died long before. She enjoyed those even though they were confusing. Margaret Thatcher, former Prime Minister of the United Kingdom, also suffered from dementia. The biographic film about her final years, *Iron Lady,* did a wonderful job of illustrating her frequent "conversations" with her deceased husband, Denis.[32] These were portrayed as sweet times for Mrs. Thatcher, giving her a chance to sort through her emotions.

Since I wasn't prepared for Nana's nightmares and hallucinations, I wrongly thought she was making stories up to frustrate me or be difficult. As a result, I lost the opportunity to hold her close and comfort her. Watch for this to happen and be ready to help your loved one work through their fears and confusion.

Look for the Blessing in Change

I've lived my entire life in the Midwest where we enjoy the most beautiful of God's gifts— four seasons. I not only look forward to the rhythm of creation, I crave it. The colors and smells. The way 50° in spring brings out my t-shirts, and the same temperature in November, my sweaters—the birth, and rebirth, of flowers in March. The death of leaves in October.

It's all change, and it's good if you see it with open eyes, ears, mind, and heart. Your perspective affects every part of this journey. Will you maximize your time together, to grow through the experience . . . or waste this opportunity, this gift, of time and focus?

"People say, when you have children, everything changes. But maybe things are awakened that were already there." - Meryl Streep

Summary Points

- Change is either good or bad—rarely indifferent. Which one you experience is mainly decided by your perspective. It's hard—extremely hard. But work to stay positive.

- Some changes are subtle and adapting can be as simple as applying a dose of encouragement, moving a rug, or keeping a list.

- Other changes may seem to suck the life out of you. That's when you'll need enough courage for both you and your loved one.

These changes will require your patience, above all else. That sense of humor I keep mentioning, and courage, are critical for you to exercise. Why? Tough decisions are on the horizon. The time is coming—soon—when you'll need to add others to their direct care.

Chapter 11

Optimism Paves the
Path to Personal Growth

"You'll miss the best things if you keep your eyes shut."
- DR. SEUSS

Glass half-full. Glass half-empty. We tend to experience life from one of these two points of view. Your choice impacts everything you do and say, how you handle good times, and bad.

I am a glass half-full person. I always have been and always will (unless developing dementia flips that on me).

Glass half-empty folks might say I am unrealistic. A Pollyanna, naive and unwilling to look truth square in the eye.

I would respond that they are self-defeatists. Unwilling to believe in the potential of others to lift situations; too eager to give up rather than do the hard work of finding a solution. Or creating one.

A Positive Perspective Can Be Our Lifeline

I'll admit it—I love Hallmark movies. They are glass half-full stories, full of optimism and hope. My sons tease me about this addiction, a lot. But these films encourage me and illustrate our positive traits, and our striving for good. The villain is reformed, the lost loves find each other, and challenges are solved. What's not to love about that (says the glass half-full gal)?

> *If, through this journey, we're to move beyond mere survival to personal growth, you need a glass half-full perspective. You may not be able to count on me for optimism—I have no idea what my perspective will be in the middle and late stages of my dementia.*
>
> *Ha—my dementia. What a funny thing to say. As if I own this disease when we both know it fully owns me. Which illustrates this point: you must be in control, but let me believe that I am, so I cooperate rather than fight you at every turn. It's a matter of respect. You'll need to encourage me a lot—gently pushing me, firmly pulling, quietly nudging. Whatever it takes to make progress toward our daily goal. And it's important I have a daily goal.*

You'll need a lot of encouragement during this caregiving journey, too, from the community you build, from family and friends. Kind people will ask how you are doing, how your loved one is doing. But they won't truly get it, can't completely understand, unless they've walked this path. You will be so thankful to have a support village.

Optimism = Longer, Healthier Life

Data abounds supporting the health benefits of positivity. Looking to the bright side, seeing the silver lining, walking on the sunny side—just a few of the many idioms to say positive thinking improves, even extends, our life.

Researchers at the Mayo Clinic list several health benefits that may occur from optimism and positive thinking.[33]

- Increased life span
- Lower rates of depression
- Lower levels of distress
- Greater resistance to the common cold
- Better psychological and physical well-being
- Better cardiovascular health and reduced risk of death from cardiovascular disease
- Better coping skills during hardships and times of stress

Scientists aren't sure why positive people experience these health benefits. Maybe it's because optimism helps us cope better with stress, which we all know is a health killer. Maybe because positive people generally live healthier lifestyles . . . better diet, more exercise, less bad habit excesses.

It Takes Patience, Acceptance, and Respect

So, how do you get and give enough encouragement to fill up your anti-frustration tank? By more than getting encouragement or ignoring problems. I'll illustrate this through the 2012 film, *Quartet*, starring Maggie Smith and Billy Connolly.[34]

This sweet film is the story of a retirement home for professional musicians and the residents' efforts to organize a fundraising event. Not to knock artistic folks, but they can be a competitive bunch, and this tendency is clearly shown among the home residents. It's humorous to watch octogenarians try to one-up each other about how big a star they were, how well they can perform now, and who had the most shocking affairs.

Maggie Smith is new resident, Jean—a former superstar—who was once married to another resident. There was quite a scandal when they split decades prior, and Jean's arrival causes a community hubbub. Friends convince Jean and three others, including her ex-husband, to recreate their infamous vocal quartet from the opera, "Rigoletto." What follows are the requisite personal attacks, misunderstandings, and reconciliations.

What's most touching is how the residents handle Cissy, one of the quartet members who has dementia. Her friends show patience, acceptance, respect, and when needed, redirection, without any hint of condescension. When Cissy seems mentally lost or on a tangent, they divert her to another reasonable reality to get her back on track. They're not demeaning or frustrated by her slow nature. They love her as she is, understand the changes she has experienced, and help guide her safely through each day.

Notice what I said: patience, acceptance, respect.

People say parenting isn't for cowards. This is true. Why? Because there's no comprehensive instruction manual that applies to every situation and unique child. The same can be said for dementia care.

So, you should focus on a few key goals. All else will fall in line and be given the right priority if you weigh everything against these points: being patient, limiting frustration, accepting me fully in whatever phase I am in, and making sure you and anyone else treat me with respect.

In caring for Nana, I learned how to encourage both of us. Many of these efforts created special memories for me and led us to grow together during the journey. Understand that this is a hard, tough road, and I'm not trying to diminish that reality. But it's all about their quality of life. Don't mourn what is lost. Focus on what is possible.

More Picasso than Monet

Nana attended an adult daycare for two months. When I picked her up one Thursday, I noticed she had this mischievous grin on her face. She carried a large canvas in her arms and excitedly declared she had a surprise for me. Careful to hide the front until we arrived home, her enthusiasm was so cute. She was a sports gal to the core—softball, basketball. Artsy things were my arena, not hers. Other than her ceramics phase while my dad was in the Air Force stationed on Guam, and she was trying to keep busy, I never knew her to "make" anything.

Once inside our house, she joyfully handed me her gift: a 16'x16' oil painting on white canvas. A first for her, no doubt, and she seemed quite proud of it. I would try to describe her masterpiece, but I think it's best to let you enjoy it for yourself.

I was smart enough not to attempt a guess at her design—I have made that classic parenting mistake before, more than once.

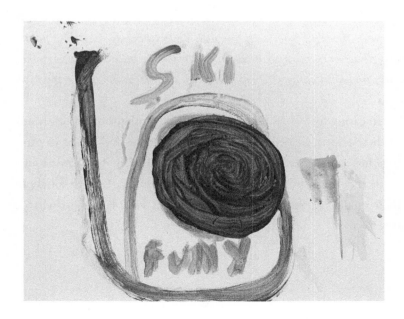

"Mom, this is amazing! Tell me about it," I said with hesitation and big eyes.

I should have known to expect the unexpected from this lady. She responded, rather irritated, "Well, can't you tell what it is?"

Ugh, my tactic failed. So, I gave it my best shot. "Someone is skiing, and they are wearing purple and look funny."

"The skier went down and then in circles! I picked purple because that's your favorite color. I didn't know what to paint, and this is how it ended up. I thought it looked silly, so I just added that 'funy' in at the end. It's not very good, so do with it what you want."

She was rarely indecisive, so I never heard her true thoughts about the work, which we simply titled "Purple Skier." I do know she enjoyed the activity, doing something new and out of her wheelhouse. Her daycare folks said she was chatty the entire time, talking with and helping the other guests who were not quite as coherent as she was, laughing and making jokes. Much better engagement than usual.

I mentioned the painting in our conversations over the next few days to get as much mental mileage out of it as possible. We talked about the painting subject, how she held the brush, if she enjoyed making it, how this compared to making her ceramic nativity on Guam (she could remember stuff from the 1960s pretty well) . . . as much as I could pull out of her experience.

Periodically, I uncovered her artwork and we talked about it again since she didn't recall having painted it. This helped her connect, talk, and to think.

Time Is the Greatest Gift of All

I've already said you will need to spend time with me to track my disease progression and know how to guide me and care for me. That's the practical perspective. The growing, loving perspective I need is based on my reality—I won't have a lot of time left.

Yes, it can take years for dementia to complete its damage. Or it can take months. So many factors will affect my remaining time, and let's face it, no one knows how many days we have, anyway.

Nana and I had lunch together every Saturday at a local deli. It took us about 2 hours to eat, mostly due to me, not her, because I would talk a lot and have always been a slow eater. For a while after her diagnosis, this outing continued normally. Eventually, she began to eat less, but still enjoyed being around other people.

Once she moved to a rehab facility, every Saturday I brought that same deli lunch to her, and we would eat together. She didn't necessarily recognize our meal, thinking it was food from a new place, but she certainly enjoyed it.

There were a few weeks when she simply wasn't interested in eating and wouldn't engage. One of my best decisions was to adapt instead of getting frustrated or angry. I bought less food, and we ate in her room. Later, I only brought lunch for me, we ate in her room, and she snacked on her beloved Pringles. Learn to go with the flow.

So, let's avoid later regrets for you and make the sacrifices to spend time together while we can. Intentional, simple, meaningful time. Making memories, yes, mostly for you, but
I will enjoy it all.

A word about perspective in this—plan out memories. People don't normally do that. We plan trips, plan activities, plan events. But do we carefully consider the impact those will have on our lives, on who we are, or who we are becoming? Memories, not simply activities, must be intentional.

Schedule lunches that I can see on my calendar. Plan simple activities for us to enjoy together. Read to me, or me to you while I can, and work together on making dinner, folding laundry, or taking walks.

Make sure I have a porch swing, glider rocker, rocking recliner . . . or all of them. I love to rock and swing, but I must be safe. We can watch musicals (I love musicals), listen to music, and talk about it, or chat about the news of the day. Visit museums, shop together, or go to a concert. It's okay that I might not remember our activities. I'll remember feeling loved.

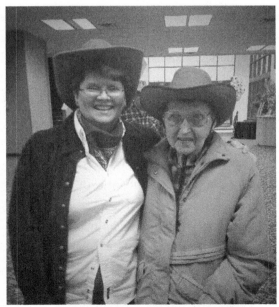

Me and Nana at a school fundraising auction – she loved events like that.

LIFE GIVING DEMENTIA CARE

The future companion workbook offers more ideas. Just understand their capabilities and interest will wane at some point, and you should adjust as needed. Please, keep moving forward. Standing still is basically moving backward. Your time together can be special, regardless of their abilities. Keep a perspective of optimism, of the glass always half-full. Like Dory says in the Disney film, *Finding Nemo*, "Just keep swimming, swimming, swimming!"

Remember That I Can't . . . Wait, What Did I Say?

You've been there. Talking to a friend, you start to describe a former mutual co-worker you bumped into recently. The three of you worked together for over ten years. For the life of you, their name is lost. Totally slips your mind. The train has left the station. It's maddening, isn't it?

People used to say forgetfulness began in our 60's. In recent years that has been revised to around age forty-five. (Makes you feel better, doesn't it—you're just getting older.) The problem seems more challenging with names for most people. Why is that? Why names and not faces?

According to a 2017 blog titled "4 Reasons Why We Forget People's Names" in *Psychology Today*, we remember faces because they are visually based, associated with events or other people, and our brains are basically wired to remember.[35] We recall words in general because we can usually come up with a synonym if our first choice fails to surface in conversation.

Names, though, are a different animal. They are generally arbitrary, don't have substitutes, often can be longer or multiworded, and in the grand scheme of talking, we use names far less than most other words. The odds are stacked against us.

For a dementia patient, this challenge is ample. I mean

ambivalent. No, wait . . . I mean it's amplified or something like that. Get the point?

I'll forget more than names and words. I'll forget comments, even entire conversations. And if my body outlives my mind, I will forget faces, too. This will become a major source of frustration for both of us, so it is important to get in front of this by preparing yourself and my close circle. You can't prepare me—I won't remember. But it'll comfort me to discuss early on that you are ready to handle this, because I'll worry about that.

There are two key points here. First, expect them to forget. Earlier, I suggested that the expectation bar needs to be set low for anything related to memory but higher for your interaction and engagement. Err on the side of them forgetting.

The second point is this: when they forget, don't repeat the information, tacking on the phrase, "Don't you remember?" Also on the naughty list is, "I already told you" and "We've talked about this three times already!" If I remembered, I wouldn't be asking again.

These statements don't help anyone. Saying these make them feel badly, you feel guilty, and whatever you were talking about gets lost in the shuffle. The only time it's right to use the phrase "do you remember" is if you're talking about something that happened at least 20 years prior.

As your loved one starts to lose names and faces, a well-labeled family photo book comes in handy. Flip through stacks of pictures. You can make (or commission from a crafty friend) an online scrapbook. There are also innovative products available to help them with most things—hearing, remembering, doing simple things as their coordination declines. Do your research. There are resources included in the appendix.

I took the online route and made a book using Shutterfly.[36] There are several online photo book companies, and most of the time at least one of them has a sale going. I uploaded digital photos and took phone pictures of prints I knew Nana would enjoy but that were taken pre-digital. Then I added text to give the people's names, relationship to Nana, and where/what was happening in the picture. Looking at this album became one of our favorite "together" activities, and I often caught her looking at it one her own. This idea is a winner.

Encouragement comes in many shapes and sizes. You will spend lots of time together, whether by necessity or design, so it makes sense to be intentional about how that time is spent. You absolutely can have fun. It's all about quality of life. Their life, and yours. We all want higher quality, right? There's a 1944 song sung by Bing Crosby that says it all. Here's the first part.

"Ac-Cent-Tchu-Ate the Positive"[37] (Harold Arlen, music; Johnny Mercer, lyrics)

> *You've got to ac-cent-tchu-ate the positive*
> *E-lim-i-nate the negative*
> *Latch on to the affirmative*
> *Don't mess with Mister In-Between*
> *You've got to spread joy up to the maximum*
> *Bring gloom down to the minimum*
> *Have faith, or pandemonium*
> *Liable to walk upon the scene*

Summary Points

- Search for ways to encourage them and you. Encouragement is like clear, cool water for the parched soul.

- Optimism is totally possible on this journey, and worthwhile. This doesn't mean denying the inevitable; it's believing today will bring something new. Growth comes from new things.

- Intentionally plan "new" into days—it stretches them, and that will buy you more enjoyable time. Use the time gained to your benefit and to help encourage others.

- Plan activities that bring happiness. Your loved one won't remember what you did, but they will remember the feeling.

Encouragement, optimism, positivity—all terms that simply mean you need to create ways for both of you to look forward to each new day. Let's be realistic—this will not be easy. It's hard, draining work and can be all-consuming. You can win this battle by anticipating when it will come, knowing what it looks like, and understanding what to do.

Chapter 12

The Things You Forget

"The most painful thing is losing yourself in the process of loving someone too much, and forgetting that you are special, too."
- ERNEST HEMMINGWAY

Stressed, distressed, anxious, burdened, uptight . . . lost.

In the article "Stress in America 2019," published by the American Psychological Association, it was noted that while general stress levels have remained fairly constant, the percentage of people experiencing stress is rising.[38] Political and social unrest, affordable and accessible health care, mass shootings, climate change, safety, and financial security are all issues that stress us out. The specific issues may change each year, but stress is real.

What happens when, on top of "life," you add becoming a dementia caregiver? You might forget to consider other people or fail to remember important events. You may forget who you are as a person.

Perhaps this is common sense, but an Alzheimer's Association web article about caregiver stress states caring for a loved one with dementia can be overwhelming and create high levels of stress.[39] Trust me—you may be much more stressed than you realize.

The article lists 10 signs you have caregiver stress, including denial, anger, depression, sleeplessness (and the resulting health problems), among others. Included are great tips for managing them, like getting support from others, relaxation techniques, physical activity, and being uber intentional about self-care. All valuable suggestions you should follow.

Be sure to include groups like the Alzheimer's Association in your care community—they are tremendous resources. But I don't just want to tell you things to remember—I also want to warn you about the things you may forget.

Forgetting Your Priorities

NFL Hall of Fame running back, Gale Sayers said, "The Lord is first, my friends are second, and **I am third**."[40] He set, very clearly, the relational priorities in his life. This is both inspirational and honest. Sayers lived his life this way.

If I had to make a similar list about my caregiver time, it would look something like this: "My caregiving is first, my job is second, my kids are third, the Lord is third and a half, my friends are fourth, I am fifth . . . oh, and my husband is somewhere in there."

I'm ashamed and embarrassed by this. I didn't mean for it to happen, and I wouldn't encourage this order of priorities for anyone, at any time. Out-of-whack priorities sneak up on you, slowly, but surely. At the time, I would have vehemently denied this was my reality if you had pointed it out.

I didn't realize the state of my life at that time until about a year after Nana passed. Little side comments spoken by a coworker, an observation from family about changes in my behavior or responses, a friend's expression when I didn't remember their big events—I started noticing things. I wish someone would have forced me to recognize my tunnel vision, that I was only seeing my caregiver role. Instead, I left everyone and everything else behind in some way.

After caregiving and work, I had nothing left. Not time. Not energy of any kind, physical or emotional. Everyone in my life suffered, even the one I was caring for—Nana.

Forgetting Family and Friends

Here's how bad it became during the months before and after her death in April of 2016.

In February of 2017, a cousin contacted me that my uncle, her dad, was in a rehab hospital. During that conversation I asked if she knew how our Uncle JR was doing. Stunned, she asked, "Don't you know he died last fall?"

Wow. I was heartbroken that no one had contacted me about this, and I cried sporadically about it for days. I was devastated that I was so blatantly overlooked by my family and unable to pay my respects.

It's important to me that I remember my loved ones who've passed, so I opened my phone calendar to enter his death date event. That's when I saw it—his funeral was already in my calendar. Travel reminders, notes . . . everything.

Not only did I know about his death, I had actually attended his funeral in Illinois. For two days.

This realization caused me more anguish than the "news" of his death. I couldn't believe I forgot something like that. How could I be so out of touch, so distracted, so *anything* to completely forget an uncle's death and funeral? That was a huge wakeup call for me and lead to serious self-evaluation.

Whether you plan to hold life's hand rather than be dragged down the street, my priorities may push aside everything else in your life. To minimize this (note I didn't say to prevent), you should intentionally make plans that will protect your priorities. This won't happen by accident. Be creative and be flexible. I love that you are caring for me.

But I don't want you to get lost in the process. You are important to me, so take care of yourself, too.

Here's the catch: Most of the people in your life honestly won't understand the priorities tension you'll feel.

They'll know you are busier as a caregiver, that there are financial and time pressures. They may understand you have new and constant frustrations, and your relationships may be strained. Folks generally aren't blind or foolish. But for the realities of caregiving? Most folks are clueless. So set realistic expectations of your "people." Those closest to you will do the challenging work of learning and supporting you in ways you won't think to ask.

Forgetting Your Work

Work and career are such big parts of our lives. According to the U.S. Bureau of Labor Statistics, in 2018 American workers averaged 8.5 hours per week day and 5.4 hours per weekend day.[41] Our productivity has increased 400% since 1950. We work a lot.

It may seem counterintuitive to warn that you may forget your work during this journey. But think about the stress we've already discussed, and its profound impact on your health. It will be nearly impossible to avoid this affecting your work.

I was fortunate to be working at a faith-based organization with a boss that understood my caregiver challenges, to a degree. As long as my work was completed, I was allowed full schedule flexibility. On days that Nana required my full attention, I would occasionally take a PTO or vacation day.

Flexibility at work, while very generous and absolutely needed, contributed to my forgetting things. Medical visits, planned activities, research—the frequent disruption in my train of thought and project work led me to drop the ball at times. Had it not been for the tremendous support from my assistants and co-workers, I probably would have either been fired or given a "put up or shut up" ultimatum. Even the most patient of bosses would not tolerate a lengthy period of nonproductivity.

Several strategies can help minimize the impact caregiving has on your work; these can help you continue feeling good about your caregiver efforts, while helping to preserve your career path and work relationships.

- Be discerning in choosing your employer, whether you ever become a caregiver or not. Invest your precious, limited lifetime with an organization that values you and what you do.
- Communicate clearly, honestly, and often with those around you. I'm not suggesting you whine or complain. But block out caregiving time commitments on your work calendar. Plan around those events. Make sure subordinates and supervisors are aware. Allow them to help, to pray for you, and to step in and cover when needed. My assistant left notes reminding me to drink the water sitting right there on my desk because I would forget. Others, on their own, often took on my responsibilities without my asking because I didn't try to hide my challenges.
- Be organized. Make lists . . . and *follow* them. I was good at making a list and putting events on my calendar. But then I wouldn't check either and ended up forgetting important activities or meetings.
- Make appointments with yourself to check projects or specific work goal progress. Schedule time with co-workers to catch up both personally and work wise. *Be intentional.*

If you are open and honest—transparent—most people will be kinder and more supportive than you can imagine. I believe folks want to help and, if given the opportunity, will rise to the occasion. Be wise enough to say you need help, and humble enough to accept it.

Forgetting Yourself

In the 1960s to 1970s, the social battle cry among younger adults was to "find yourself." Many turned to drugs, alcohol, or communal living to figure out who they were as a person—doing anything they could that was anti-cultural. This focus hasn't changed, much. As I write this in 2020, the Millennial and Gen Z members (born 1980–2015) are still trying to understand themselves. They often take a gap year after high school or make a habit of job hopping.

Self-awareness is crucial to maturity. Understanding yourself provides a foundation that is tough to topple. But I promise you— being a caregiver will rock your world, and anyone close enough will feel the quake.

Three months after Nana's death, I had my annual work review. The prior two years had been rough. My boss asked how I was doing now that life had changed dramatically for me. As I struggled to craft a semi-coherent response, a moment of clarity hit me. I didn't have a clear basis to evaluate how I was doing. I couldn't remember what I used to be like, how I behaved or related to others, pre-caregiving.

How did this hit me? Have you ever picked up a glass of what you expected to be milk and quickly realized it was orange juice? Startled by the reality, unable to hold your reaction, completely disappointed and unsure of what to do next? That summarizes how I felt. Total disorientation.

Realizing that I not only had veered way away from "me," but I couldn't remember when or how it happened . . . I was angry, scared, and completely unsure of how to fix it.

Of all the ways being a caregiver affected me, this was the biggest, and it was both negative and positive. Negative in that my loss of self and awareness of others, my temporary tunnel vision, caused me to miss out on life in so many ways. It became more difficult for people to be around me because "silver lining" me became a complainer, a Negative Nellie; so completely out of my territory, and I never even noticed.

In the end, though, it was a positive impact. I realized that I never truly understood who I was. It was tough, often painful work to dig into "me" and my experiences, to figure out who I was so I could return—maybe even a new and improved version.

After years of self-evaluation and reflection, of thoughtful conversation with friends and family, I am finally close to the better parts of who I was before being a caregiver. I've grown in many ways and have achieved a goal I never knew I needed—I believe I have finally found myself.

I share these details because I want you to understand—losing yourself on this journey is not just a possibility; it's a probability. Yet, it doesn't need to be a personal setback. Use this experience for personal growth. Don't walk this path alone—take your people along for the ride.

What's the Answer for You?

Having cared full time for my mother, and part time for my father, I've learned a thing or two. For one, I'm in good company. According to caregiveraction.org, in 2009, over 65 million people, 29% of the U.S. population, were caring for a loved one.[42] This statistic will certainly keep climbing.

So, what should you know about protecting your life while you share it as a caregiver?

- Don't underestimate the high cost of rushing past the other people in your world in your quest to take care of your loved one. Be intentional about your relationships.
- Talk to family and friends about your struggles when you can—they will feel wanted and useful and you'd be surprised at their wisdom. At this point, they'll remember more about being your age than about being their own.
- Look for encouragement—it will come from unexpected places. Nana's medical folks often complimented me on how I cared for her. It lifted my spirits, especially on days I felt like an ogre for having lost my patience with her.
- Develop the habit of journaling. You don't need to author a novel every day. Use the bullet method or digital tools—whatever works. Just get started. Spilling your innermost thoughts and feelings, struggles and joys, onto the blank page will free your mind and give you a trail of where you've been to help you better enjoy where you are going.
- Talk to someone(s) who gets it. The doctor, a support group, a friend who's been there and done this. A counselor. Letting things build in your mind benefits no one.

No solution is one-size-fits-all. What worked for me and Nana may or may not work for you and your loved one, or for others. Keep trying, though. Watch for new, innovative ideas, and use your personal and online resources. There's usually a way to resolve problems.

Summary Points

- It is no surprise that being a caregiver is stressful. Learn to recognize the stress signs so you can address personal issues quickly and completely.

- Caregiving is all-consuming. Monitor your priorities carefully, and immediately take steps to right your ship as needed.

- It's easy to leave family, friends, work—even yourself—behind as you focus on your loved one. Please be intentional to communicate well, and often, with others. Find people who truly understand what you are experiencing. Don't feel fear or shame, especially with those who know and love you.

- There's so much opportunity to grow as a person through caregiving. Don't waste it.

For us to successfully walk through my illness, it's vital that you stay grounded in who you are and who and what is most important. Yes, you will spend a lot of time caring for me, and priorities may be skewed at times. But I am leaving; you have the rest of your life. Focus on the bigger picture. If you do, you'll be equipped to make tough care decisions that are coming soon.

Chapter 13

Adult Day Care Can Be a Great Option—But Buyer Beware

"I don't subscribe to the thesis, 'Let the buyer beware,' I prefer the disregarded one that goes, 'Let the seller be honest.'"
- ISAAC ASIMOV

On Thursday, January 15, 2015 at 3 p.m., I received a call from a physician at my dad's rehab hospital reporting his vital signs were unexpectedly fluctuating. They were monitoring him closely—no cause for concern, but they wanted me to be aware. Nana and I had visited him that morning after her kidney checkup. He was a bit quiet but was upbeat and seemed to be continuing his recovery trajectory. So, the call surprised me.

Six hours later, my cell rang again. It was a hospital resident calling to report my dad was "crashing"—what did I want them to do? What? Dad had a DNR (Do Not Resuscitate) order in place, so why ask me this? My dad documented his instructions to die rather than live on a ventilator. Shocked and disoriented, I said I would call him back so I could talk with my husband. That probably was the resident's turn to think, "What?" Call him back while my dad was fighting for his life?

My husband called back immediately, getting the same report, so he reminded them of the DNR. Racing to the hospital 20 minutes away (we made it in 10), we arrived to see the nurse carrying a large trash bag of medical paraphernalia out of my dad's room. He died five minutes earlier. Ignoring his DNR, the medical staff intubated him, but he didn't survive.

We arrived back home around 1 a.m. Nana was asleep and didn't know we had raced to the hospital, so I decided to wait until the next morning to tell her the news. After she was up and dressed, I carefully explained the sequence of events and that dad died. She clearly followed my words and was heartbroken at the news.

The next day we began funeral arrangements. (My parents had no plans in place, other than owning graves in Illinois that we will never use, and I can't seem to sell). Through the days leading to the services, I'd have to say she was pretty upbeat—not completely surprising since folks typically launch into "things to do" mode in those situations.

Connecting the Dots

Over the following weeks, Nana's demeanor didn't change. I knew she missed my dad desperately; they were married for nearly 60 years. Other than an occasional 15-second burst of tears, she was rarely sad, often forgot he was gone, and seemed emotionally steady—certainly more than the rest of us. Her health was stable, medical checkups continued to be social events for her, and her cognitive function seemed to improve slightly. A rebirth, of sorts.

This was definitely a surprise until my research helped connect the dots. What we were experiencing was almost a perfect storm. Her cognitive decline was such that, while her pain from losing my dad was very real . . . it was also very fleeting. She couldn't remember her loss long enough to be terribly sad. Contributing to this was the fact that, after getting her breakfast each morning, my dad would normally descend to his workshop in our basement until bedtime. Nana's improved health was mainly a result of timing. Dad had been hospitalized for many weeks, and she was no longer worrying about him. Her meds were working, and her new treatment regimen of taking two different, but complementary, meds was helping slow her mental decline.

After a few months, though, her spirits began to dip. She was less engaged and sort of disinterested. Naturally, I attributed this to her disease. But in hindsight, I should have realized she might have been lonely. At the time, it didn't occur to me. Three other people lived with her, one of whom was home 24/7 managing his own business. We still had one son at home, in high school, so folks were always running in and out. We saw her, talked to her, tried to engage her daily. How could she possibly be lonely?

In fact, she was. It is quite common for dementia patients to feel isolated and lonely. They have probably lost friends, maybe to this or other illnesses. They have diminished freedom and decision-making ability. Friends may be uncomfortable coming around. Nana's good friend from work only visited once after her diagnosis. Once. She said she couldn't bear seeing Nana "this way," not the friend she once knew. How sad.

Nana was lonely, and I knew I couldn't let that continue or get worse. There's a lot of research on the negative health impact of loneliness, but the pain is especially strong for dementia patients. Nana's gerontologist suggested we involve professional care and explore adult day care. That could give Nana purpose, relationships, and activity—opportunity to learn something new, stretching her brain a bit.

Do Your Daycare Research

Adult day care facilities come in many shapes and sizes, run well or poorly, by people of integrity . . . and not. After talking with our doctors to get their insight and referrals, I selected four centers to visit. They could not have been more different. Kind of like *Goldilocks and the Three Bears*, they ranged from shameful to fabulous. I am eternally grateful one was fabulous.

You should ask certain key questions when you interview day care managers. Facilities, staffing, and finances are all topics to discuss. I will share a more comprehensive list of considerations in the planned companion workbook.

One center was in an office park. As I drove up, I could see through the windows that folks were sitting around doing basically nothing, staring blankly at the TV or floor. No staff in sight, and too many folks in that one area. I drove past. There was *no way* I would take Nana there.

The second and third centers were nice enough. The staff, in admissions anyway, were kind and helpful. They seemed to answer my questions fully, though in hindsight my preparation for these visits was sorely lacking. Sometimes you don't know what you don't know. I took pictures and notes on each visit; I recommend you do both at any facility you visit. I didn't talk with clients, but I did watch their activities and demeanor, informally assessing their dementia level as best I could. One of the centers seemed a solid contender, but online reviews were concerning.

You'll Know When It Fits

A friend who knew about Nana's disease suggested I visit Joy's House.[43] Her mom was a client for a couple of years and loved it so much that my friend's husband joined their board of directors. That's a high recommendation, so I scheduled a visit. What an incredible difference compared to the other centers—head and shoulders above!

I later took Nana for a visit, then a trial day. She fought the idea, of course. The comfort of her bedroom, rocker, and TV had become a little too appealing. Plus, the idea of a day care center meant she needed care, someone to help. She never genuinely accepted her need for personal aid until well into the late stage of her illness.

Despite my complaints and fears, I started attending the day care center. Eventually I had to admit how much I enjoyed my weekly visits. I was free to make crafts, sing songs, even watch TV or rest in a recliner. Joy's House was built like a big, sprawling home. The staff was so kind to us, and I joked with the other folks, who were mostly like me. They called me "Miss Lois." Yes, some folks didn't, or couldn't, chat or do activities. But I felt safe, cared for, and comfortable. That's the most important thing when you choose others to help care for me.

Strong centers should give you a daily report so you can monitor your loved one's experience. Joy's House was great at that. I wanted Nana's perspective too and always asked her to share about her day. But getting her thoughts was just like trying to pull information out of a teenager, but with worse results.

"Mom, how was your day today?" I'd ask as we drove home.

Her reply was pretty consistent, I'll give her that much. "Eh, so so. I won't complain."

Her daily experience reports listing her activities, demeanor, and interactions . . . often with photos . . . told the real story. She was usually smiling, laughing, and happy. She could give me any report she wanted, but I knew better. Miss Lois was a huge hit—they loved her, and she loved her center!

Choosing a Daycare

Of course, you can hire someone to stay with and engage your loved one at home. That choice comes with its own set of concerns. But if you decide to engage an adult day care, here are a few of the top points you should consider.

- Philosophy of care—is it individual or group focused?
- Is it a medical or non-medical model?
- What is their licensure, staff qualifications, training, and turnover?
- Facility safety and cleanliness (does it smell bad, odd, or overtly like Lysol)?
- What is the type, frequency, and pattern of activities?
- Do they celebrate their guests in any way—individual or holiday parties?
- What is the cost, how do you pay, are there scholarships, and is outside funding available?
- How do they protect their guests from leaving unattended (aka wandering)?
- How do they handle health events during the day?
- What reporting do they provide to licensing authorities and to you?
- Can they expel a guest, and can you withdraw at any time?
- Do they offer any type of support to you as a caregiver, such as respite days, a blog, newsletters, and such?

We were very blessed that Nana's dementia level fit within Joy's House care ability and that she received a scholarship to help us afford a few days each week. It took about a month to select a center, enroll, and begin attending, so plan accordingly and do your research well before the need for daycare. We moved quickly, so you might need more time than we took. I never had to select a childcare facility for my sons (Nana babysat for them), but if you have been through that process, this will seem familiar. If you research, check online reviews carefully, and ask for references and call them, the process can run smoothly.

A lot is at stake in this decision, and you should track the disease progress carefully. One day an adult day care center will no longer fill the gap for them. One day it will be necessary to take the next step to engage a higher level of aid.

Summary Points

- To know when it's time to involve others in routine care, you'll need to connect the dots on everything about your loved one. It's not likely they'll tell you it's time or ask for a nurse or daycare.

- Adult daycare can be awful and depressing, or uplifting and amazing. Do lots of research ahead of time. Visit your top candidates at different times of the day, talk to other involved families, and consult with folks who have been down this road.

- Don't expect them to skip happily to their first day. But they'll come around if it's a good decision and you've chosen the right center. If they don't, pay close attention and investigate. Fight the temptation to dismiss their feelings or comments. They may not recall the details, but they will know how they feel.

Once I began to add professional caregivers into the mix, it meant Nana was entering the late stage of her disease. The decisions you will soon make are a bit less complex in some ways but carry far more weight—from here on out it's more difficult to reverse course.

Part III

The Last Stage

Chapter 14

In-Home or Out—Where to Live

"Home is where, when you have to go there, they have to take you in."
- ROBERT FROST

Consider these 2015–2017 caregiver statistics from the U.S. Department of Health and Human Services, Center for Disease Control.[44]

- 1 in 5 adults provided regular care or aid to a friend or family member with health issues.
- Nearly half of those folks have provided care for at least two years.
- Almost a third supplied care for at least 20 hours per month.
- 58% of caregivers were women, 19% were age 65 or older, and 1 in 3 were caring for a parent or parent-in-law.
- 80% managed household tasks and over half supplied personal care.

According to the 2018 study, "Aging in Place in America," commissioned by Clarity and The EAR Foundation, senior citizens today fear moving into a nursing home and losing their independence more than they fear death.[45] Nana was definitely in this camp. I can't remember the number of times she declared, "Do not *ever* put me in a nursing home—I'll disown you!"

After her dementia diagnosis, I would jokingly respond that I wouldn't have to as long as she didn't break her hip, or something big like that. She always viewed herself as invincible, so this was my way to encourage her to be careful. In the end, the nursing home decision was made for us.

On Christmas day in 2015, she broke her hip. We think she fell around 5:00 a.m. trying to reach her walker for a potty visit, but we didn't find her until 9:00 that morning. It was an unbelievably long, difficult day. My husband and I managed to return home from the hospital around 10:00 p.m. to open presents with our family (who had waited all day for us), then returned to the hospital for her midnight surgery.

The surgery went very well—she was a tough, tough lady—and her rehab began the next day. Four days later, on her eighty-eighth birthday, she was discharged to a rehab nursing facility. I never used the term *nursing home* with her even though that's actually what it was. Her rehab progressed extremely well, and it looked like she might get to come home in a few weeks, which was a huge, but incredibly happy, surprise for us.

She experienced a setback when a stent in her left thigh artery completely blocked. She developed sores on her lower leg, the toes turned black, and the pain was beyond even her high tolerance. Since this was already her third stent, replacing it was not an option. Either we allowed gangrene to set in, or we amputated.

I knew amputation meant she would probably never return home. We had neither the resources nor ability to supply the necessary care. My discussion with her about this was amazingly short. Her pain was so high, she said, "Just cut it off. I can't take it anymore!" We couldn't tell her amputating meant this facility would be her new home. She wouldn't understand or remember any explanation I might offer. She asked me often to take her home, and I had to either change the subject, distract her, or outright lie.

On Valentine's Day, 2016, her left leg was amputated mid-thigh. In typical Nana fashion, she managed the surgery quite well, and her healing was rapid. But this was more evidence of how far her disease had progressed. The pre-dementia Nana would never, *ever*, have allowed her leg to be amputated. The loss of personal freedom and mobility would have been too humiliating for her.

But this version of Nana was different. During the months before her broken hip, she made gradual progress to accept her mental decline and resulting new normal. In December, we even Christmas shopped with her in a wheelchair. I told her the wheelchair would help her from getting too tired, and we could load all our purchases on her and the chair to help us. She was always game for helping, so the wheelchair became a tool, not an embarrassment.

Moving Nana to a nursing facility was not up for debate; the only question was for how long. We discussed the pros and cons with her, laying out plans for her recovery and return home contingent on the doctor releasing her. The doc was my ace, my willing scapegoat in keeping her in rehab when all she wanted was to go home.

It will be important that you include me in this discussion and decision. Unless I am completely unable to engage, there are creative ways to do this. You must make the effort—it's a matter of love, respect, and dignity. I've earned it. This will be hard for both of us, this new reality. But my quality of life, health, and safety need to be our priority. Ideally, we'll have this method of care conversation early in my disease, while I am more coherent. Regardless, we need to discuss it when the time comes. It just will be much easier if you can show me evidence of our prior decisions.

So, what are our care options, which should we choose, and why?

It Isn't Free

We may as well address the elephant in the room—cost. Most folks probably think home health care is less expensive than assisted living or skilled nursing care. But that's not necessarily true.

U.S. News & World Report noted that in 2018, assisted living care averaged $4,000 per month.[46] A home health aide was about 5% higher, and skilled, private nursing home care would set you back a whopping 280% more!

Compare the amount of *time* they'll need, the type of care, and the various rates. Home health aide rates averaged $150-$300 per day in 2018.[47] If they need lots of aide time, in-home care could be much more costly than an outside facility. There will be a tipping point between you managing their care, an aide, or choosing a facility away from home. Consider *all* the costs, not just monetary. If family and friends are supplying in-home care, you need to factor in the stress, coordination, and time investment. Factors can add up quickly and are significant.

Nana had a home-health aide for only five months. Amanda was scheduled for semi-weekly visits to check her vitals, answer questions, and make sure Nana was taking her meds, eating, sleeping, and toileting well. Medicare covered the cost, which was a big blessing. But our expectations and the services Nana actually received didn't always match, and it was common for visits to be cancelled or rescheduled at the last minute. If you choose this option, don't fall for a sales pitch. Read the fine print, seek out honest reviews and referrals, and hold their feet to the fire.

Payment options will vary depending on any pre-planning. Your loved one's personal assets, social security, and long-term care insurance are good options. Medicare will pay for up to 100 days in a care facility.[48] To be safe, you should plan for other funding means.

If there are no assets to speak of, government aid (Medicaid or a similar program) may be an option.

If you consider Medicaid, be aware of program eligibility rules related to assets; the rules are complex. First, understand that Medicaid is regulated at the state, not federal level. Know the rules for their state of residence.

You should also realize assets must be spent down to a stipulated level (their home is protected, generally, within certain guidelines) and they must have completely moved to a care facility in order to have a successful Medicaid application.[49] When we started Nana's application in 2016, for example, she could own no more than $1,500 in cash/savings or investments.

This can get tricky, and potentially a little frightening. To prevent folks from entering a care facility one day, giving all their money away the next, and then applying for Medicaid, the program has rules about asset transfers to others. There is a *look back* period where program authorities can review their financial information for any kind of transfers made over the prior 60 months for less than fair value (aka gifts) —big, little, birthday, wedding, charitable donations, for example. Depending on how far they dig into the weeds, and whether the gifts were made to fraudulently hide assets from Medicaid, they can delay their program eligibility, in theory, for an unlimited amount of time.

This could be devastating and eliminate key funding options. Naively, I trusted Nana's nursing home administrator to submit her Medicaid application. I followed up once, but never asked for confirmation. Six months after her death, I received a $13,500 bill in the mail for one month of care. Apparently, my state's laws allow facilities to seek reimbursement from the resident's children. Fortunately for me, the facility acknowledged that the Medicaid application was never filed—their failure—so they didn't pursue collection. To be safe, I recommend at a minimum you hire an elder law attorney to consult with you about this option and to possibly complete the application.

Your loved one probably doesn't want to be a financial burden to you or anyone. But given rising costs, there is a good chance most families will bear at least some financial burden, yours included. Make sure they have adequate life insurance pre-diagnosis to help reimburse your costs after their passing. Some policies offer an accelerated death benefit that allows policy owners to receive part of the policy face value before death. That may be an option for you.

Care at Home

One AARP survey reported that about 90% of American seniors wish to live at home for as long as possible.[50] Regardless of the circumstances, most patients prefer living at home rather than in a facility to maintain their independence.

There are multiple options to provide care at home, and the costs will vary widely depending on the level and frequency of their needs. Some of the more common options are:

- **In-home care:** Providing companionship and some transportation, doing light housekeeping, and cooking—no expected medical care
- **Home-Health care:** Includes the details above but with medical care included
- **Periodic nurse visits:** Checks their vitals, status, and well-being
- **Physical Therapist:** Provides therapy to develop balance and physical strength
- **Live-in professional:** Supplies full-time care

The clear benefits of these options, if my care level justifies it, is that I can feel safe and comfortable in my own home. I keep more independence. Often, the cost is less than moving to a care facility. But with these options, I'll require more of your time and attention—both a pro and con, depending on the circumstances. The downsides include safety: my home may be dangerous for me. I also may have to manage more of my own care, which can be risky. And unless someone is with me 24/7, my declining executive function can lead to poor decisions. This option carries a good deal of uncertainty.

Assisted Living

Shortly after Nana's diagnosis, I visited an assisted living facility owned by friends. I wasn't sure what she would need, when she would need it, or if we would be capable of providing it, so I felt it wise to start exploring options. The cost quoted at that time was about $3,200 per month for a private room. Between her social security, my dad's small pension, government aid, and my family contributing, I thought we could swing the cost if needed.

The facility was near our home, the grounds were inviting, and there were large, colorful floral arrangements everywhere. The facilities were clean, smelled fresh, were tastefully decorated, and designed with resident safety in mind. The facility offered two levels of care: minimal, with staff check-in and prescription reminders, or medium care, with a bit more medical oversight. Residents had multiple activity and excursion options, and transportation was provided for shopping, medical visits, and such. A dedicated memory care wing was under construction.

For a non-home option, it offered a real, workable choice. Nana was not interested in the least, naturally. "I don't need a nursing home!" she barked at me. I never succeeded in helping her see the difference between assisted living and a nursing home. In her mind, you were either at home or not. Let me encourage you to push through their feelings on this issue. Form over substance. Meet the goals even if the path might not be their ideal. In hindsight, I think I should have considered this more seriously for Nana.

Assisted living offers the benefits of greater personal safety, more socialization, possibly better nutrition with some medical oversight, and a proper level of independence.

The main negative is increased cost.

> *You should also realize that once I leave my home, your role will begin to shift from monitoring me to advocating for me. That can be hard to accept. It's like sending your first child off to kindergarten. You no longer know every detail of my day, all the players involved, or the conversations taking place. You'll work somewhat in the dark, so plan for it, communicate often with staff and with me. Listen to what I report and take it seriously no matter how improbable it might seem. Ask me and the staff questions. Go up the facility chain if necessary. Remember that our goal is my safety and happiness.*

I'm convinced the more you interact with facility staff, the better care your loved one will get. I generally visited Nana every other day and called her on the off days. She never heard the phone, and couldn't remember how to answer it, so I usually had to call the nurse's station to reach her. They knew I was connected and watching. It was so sad to hear them say most residents rarely had visitors or family who contacted staff.

Skilled Care Facilities, AKA Nursing Homes

There is no painless way to say this—having to move into full-time, skilled nursing care will stink if that is what our loved one needs. Having to trust strangers with their well-being, expecting them to be kind, patient, and attentive . . . these are high standards that frankly many facilities do not meet. It's like picking a daycare for your child.

U.S. News & World Report noted in 2019 that, of 546 nursing homes in my state, only 20 received a rating of 5 out of 5.[51] That's a lousy 3.7%. The odds of finding a top notch nursing home are worse than finding a needle in a haystack (which is 10%).

Fortunately, reliable independent ratings are available to help you select a skilled care facility. I'll include a list in the upcoming companion workbook. In addition to U.S News & World Report, you can check your state government resources and federal Medicare ratings. Medicare's website even includes information about past and current facility inspection deficiencies; metrics like prevalence of resident bedsores, fire safety, emergency preparedness, and food and kitchen issues are measured in detail. At the very least, this information can fuel questions for your facility interviews.

I believe the best way to choose among care options is to know me well. Talk to me, discuss options with my medical team. Absorb reputable review information, including online reviews, though you might take those with a grain of salt. The "never-satisfied" crowd can run amok with unwarranted complaints, so be discerning.

Be aware your loved one's needs will continually change. For me and Nana, her needs trajectory wasn't a steady incline, but more like climbing uneven stairs—sometimes a little bump and other times a leap, with an occasional backstep. To accommodate that reality, there are facilities offering both assisted living and skilled nursing care. The benefit is they don't have to move; they basically transfer from one wing to another. This keeps consistency in staffing and friendships. This type of facility, at least good ones, are not as common. But they exist and are a strong option.

One benefit of choosing a well-run nursing home is they will (in theory) have 24/7 care. They should be safe, have multiple engaging activity options, and receive proper medical oversight. You become freed to fully focus on your loved one and that relationship rather than deal with care details. As I said earlier, you move from monitoring to advocating. Moving Nana to a rehab facility provided me real relief and helped replace stress with memories. The negative: This may come at a prohibitive cost. The situation doesn't last forever—the average nursing home stay is two years according to the National Care Planning Council.[52] It may seem like you lose all control over their care, but that's not exactly true. Your means of control change, and you'll need to adapt. You can do this—it's all about perspective and awareness.

Hospice and Palliative Care Options

If you are like most people, when you hear the words *hospice* and *palliative* you think of cancer and the end of life. Cancer is generally the primary diagnosis of those who die in hospice care. But cardiac and dementia disease are the next two in ranking.

Let's talk about hospice and palliative care and how they differ.

Hospice care focuses on end-of-life comfort and dignity.[53] It's generally for patients who are not responding to treatment and who are expected to live six months or less. People choosing this route stop all curative efforts. The focus becomes quality of life, not quantity.

Palliative care focuses on patients with severe illness who need pain relief and symptom management. Patients are usually medically expected to survive longer than six months, contrary to hospice patients. Folks normally continue treatment efforts to cure or slow their disease. The focus is quality *and* quantity of life.

All hospice care is palliative, but not all palliative care is hospice.

Chapter 15 is dedicated to hospice and palliative care. I mention them now because they need to be considered as one of your options. Hospice and palliative care can happen at home, in a skilled care facility, and every place in between. It's not a destination as much as a philosophy that guides your decision.

Ask many questions about this part of their care. Questions like:

- How is hospice care offered and who manages it?
- Who is on the team (and is there a *team*, or is it just one person)?
- What is the care philosophy?
- How loving are the staff?
- How often and for how long is staff with each resident?
- What *exactly* does the service provide vs. what the family provides?
- What status reports are given.

It's important to know how each care option integrates hospice, because your loved one will likely need it toward the end. In 2017, the average stay for those dying in hospice (all diseases) was 76 days.[54] The average stay for those with dementia was 110 days. Nana lived in hospice care for 75 days (maybe the *only* thing that was ever average about my mom).

The Choice Is Made

You don't need to make this choice alone. Use your support community and the numerous professional and non-profit resources available. Two of the best resources I've found are Assisted Living Today [55] and Aging Care. [56] I've listed other resources in the appendix and in the planned companion workbook. Use them. Delegate research to those you trust. Follow the checklists. When you are frazzled and scared, not able to clearly think, these lists will guide your interviews and conversations.

Don't expect me to be excited about any decision, or necessarily support you. I'm sorry, but I might be downright mean and angry. Be kind, patient, and gentle with me—it's not intentional. Remember your focus questions: Am I safe, am I happy (eventually), am I pain-free? What is really most important?

Once the choice is made, and each time it is made if your loved one must move from option to option, try not to second guess yourself. This is gut-wrenching stuff, and there may be no perfect choice. Yes, moving between facilities will be traumatic for everyone, so there is an element of risk management involved with each decision.

You'll certainly feel the pain of any change far longer than your loved one will—that's a blessing in disguise of dementia. If a decision doesn't work out, or their condition worsens faster than expected causing a ramp up in care . . . it's all right. Invent an *adventure tale* to explain their moves. Be creative. It's the loving thing to do for them, and they will love the tale you weave.

Summary Points

- Most seniors' biggest fear is not death but living in a nursing home. Remember this as you make care decisions.
- Professional care is expensive. Seek experienced financial and legal counsel to navigate the options, cost, and sources of funding.
- There are several levels of care available, and needs will change over time. You may have to make care decisions multiple times.
- Make a choice and stand your ground. Don't let your loved one or others bully you, even if the decision isn't exactly popular.

It's not possible to predict when professional help will be needed, or for how long the chosen care method will be sufficient. Be aware of your loved one's ability to function, their changing wellbeing and medical needs, and make the best decisions you can *today*. That's all you can do. The day is coming, sooner than later, when you'll be faced with end-of-life choices.

Chapter 15

Is It Hospice Time?

"We cannot change the outcome, but we can affect the journey."
- ANN RICHARDSON

"Seeing death as the end of life is like seeing the horizon as the end of the ocean." - David Searles.

What's the point of these quotes? The horizon is closer than it looks; it's the beginning of the ocean, not the end. Our view is limited, a snippet of the vastness beyond. Such is death when compared to eternity.

So, let's begin this discussion with the right perspective—hospice care is the process of helping us *live* our final days on earth, to feel *loved* and to help us experience a proper *farewell* until we meet again. Hospice is not the Bataan Death March, a dreadful dirge while we wait for death. At least, it doesn't have to be.

Most dementia patients eventually need hospice care; most never receive it, either at all or not until their last days. Why?

Simply put, it's all about the rules. My doctors will decide if I qualify for hospice, and when, based on the stage of my disease progression. We are free to accept or reject that recommendation, so try to prepare—you'll make a better decision for both of us. My doctors have to predict with some level of reliability how much longer I'll live. This is harder to do than if I had cancer or heart conditions. My dementia can be unpredictable within each stage. Hospice is a big decision. Consult with several of my doctors.

Dementia presents a whole different set of challenges. Ask any dementia caregiver, on any given day, how their patient is doing. Their response can easily bounce between worse and better several times a week, even within a day. While some diseases follow a routine progression of decline in *stages*, dementia decline often changes in *inches*, with a roller coaster effect thrown in for fun.

Evidence of the patient's needs can be vague compared to many diseases. At this point, in the last stage, patients probably can't communicate their pain, wants, or desires well . . . or their needs. Caregivers must guess to some degree, including the medical community. Considering their pre-diagnosis personality can help you figure this out. Explain to the doctors how your loved one is different and when changes occurred. This is when your journal and status tracking tools will come in handy.

Watch for the Signs

In late January 2016, I received a call from Nana's nursing home. She had fallen out of bed, for the third time that month, and hit her head. Weeks before, they had placed floor pads on both sides of her bed for protection. But she still managed to miss the pad and hit the floor. This was her fourth ER visit in three weeks.

Entering her ER room, I could see she was fine, sporting a big Sponge Bob bandage on her forehead. We laughed, and I teased her about this failed nursing home escape attempt before they wheeled her off for a precautionary x-ray.

About a year earlier, shortly after my dad passed, Nana's primary care doc said that at some point her organs would start to fail, and it would probably be a train wreck when it happened due to her multiple ailments. That would be my sign to consider hospice. I naively nodded my understanding (*not!*) and carried on with life and my caregiving. I completely missed the significance of the doctor's comment. Nana, in hospice? For heaven's sake, why? I was so clueless.

Quality of Life Is Not a Cliché

Months later, with her latest fall, this was a new day. The ER doctor asked to speak with me privately. As kindly as possible, she talked about Nana's age, general condition, growing number of ailments, and the need for change in direction. Uncharacteristic for a doctor, she was beating around the bush. I rescued the situation by blurting out I knew that hospice was in our future, I just didn't know when.

"I'd pull that trigger, if I were you," she said, suddenly abandoning that bush she had been beating.

It's one thing to know in the recesses of your mind that something as final as hospice is coming; it's quite another to face it nose-to-nose. The directness of her comment was unexpected, and I was stunned.

She continued. Based on Nana's lab results, most of her organs were failing. Stage 4 kidney failure. Her COPD was worsening. Blood flow to the left leg was nonexistent, and we were probably facing amputation. We already knew the treatment to improve her bone density didn't work, so her risk of bone breaks was high. She had low blood pressure, arrhythmia, and a heart murmur, which were complicating everything. She was eighty-eight years young.

Oh, and then there was dementia driving the bus.

We reviewed medical recommendations, talked with rehab facility staff, including their supervising physician, and prayed. A lot. Nana's 60-year-old voice rang in my ears from nearly thirty years earlier, "Don't put me in a nursing home. I can't stand to just sit around and do nothing. I don't want to be a burden to you. Don't let me be dependent on anybody."

Her quality of life was terrible. Since she had no friends and leaned toward the introverted side, the facility insisted she take part in activities, even pushing her to attend group meals. Chewing was always challenging for Nana due to denture issues, and acid reflux left her esophagus scarred and narrow. To deal with this, the dining staff provided mushy food, which simply wasn't appealing to her. She preferred to eat alone, or not at all.

The day after her ER visit, we decided to transition her care to hospice.

The Same but Totally Different

The facility staff did their best to make the process simple and painless. That worked for my mom, but not for me. No matter how hard I tried to focus, to understand what the hospice intake staff was saying, all I could hear was they would help her through her final months of life. Final months.

I made the tough decision to keep her comfortable, shepherding her toward death in the way she would want. A decision that should allow me and her to spend time together, essentially carefree since others would be dedicated to her well-being. So, why was I a blooming emotional mess?

It was because I was not prepared enough ahead of time, and the staff didn't really help me manage all this beforehand, or after. So, I signed the paperwork.

I can't stress enough how important it is to learn about hospice and palliative care early in the disease's progression. To properly understand the process and full impact of care changes, you need to do your homework. Read a book or two, research online, talk to medical staff, and especially connect with support groups. I've listed some useful resources in the appendix.

Most of the care your loved one receives will seem the same as before hospice. Nana was in the same room and had basically the same nurses and routine. Actually, she *thought* she was in the same room, but wasn't. We needed her to be closer to the nurse's station for monitoring. So, one evening while she was at dinner, we moved her to a different, but identical room down the hall. I set everything up exactly as it was in her original room, and she never knew the difference.

Similarity in care was the main reason I didn't initially notice her quick, steady decline after entering hospice. Her health had been coasting for months. Other than a few quirky behavior days, and her physical therapy ending, there was little warning about what would happen over the next five weeks. I was not well prepared, and received few status updates, so how could I know?

The Nuts and Bolts of Hospice

To be blunt, signing the hospice paperwork is like signing a death warrant. Of course, doctors have already determined the body will be dying. But moving your loved one to hospice care will likely speed the process. I've been through this exercise exactly once, which doesn't inherently make me an expert. At the same time, this is a relatively small club, and members aren't exactly eager to talk about their experience. Dementia is an especially cruel disease. It offers a handful of rules with a million and one variations. No amount of study or preparation will totally prevent the surprises in store.

What are the key points you need to know as your loved one enters hospice care?

- What are their needs—emotional, medical, social?
- Are you able to meet those needs through family and friends in their home (if they're still at home), or at your home?
- If you can't meet their needs, decide if you'll hire aides or nurses to provide care, and if so, where, who, and for what time period(s).
- Is the staff specifically trained for hospice care? Is there a hospice trained physician assigned, and can your loved one's regular PCP still be involved?
- Exactly what will care include? This may seem like a silly question, but you would be surprised by the variation in care. You need to get a complete, detailed list of care to be provided and be prepared to hold the hospice staff accountable.
- How are you paying for this? The hospice admissions staff should be able to help you through this process.
- Once you sign the service forms, all efforts to prolong life will stop. Medications will focus on helping them be pain-free, comfortable, and safe. I didn't completely understand this when I signed Nana's hospice paperwork. I remember being told, repeatedly, that staff efforts would focus on keeping her comfortable. They said what they *would* do, not what they *would not* do. They would not force her to eat or drink. They would not continue her heart, kidney, and circulation medications. They would not push her to socialize or engage unless she or I specifically requested it.
- What type of status updates will you be given, how will you get them, who prepares the update, and how often?
- Who can you contact, and how, with questions about care?
- Are visitors allowed, at what times, and are you able to control that process?

Finally, understand that hospice care is final. Patients are approved for this care because they are expected to die, sooner than later. You may be tempted to think there's more time left than you really have. Don't fall for this. Plan to spend as much time with your loved one as you can.

Nana had several medical conditions, but she was stable in 2015, until her fall. Her hip surgery recovery was nothing short of miraculous for her age. Rehab was going great, for an 88-year-old. But even though she was totally bored and tired of just existing, I convinced myself she seemed content enough. I didn't realize how well her dozen daily medications coordinated to keep her alive . . . until those medications were gone.

Being totally inexperienced in the whole hospice process, I didn't connect these dots until months after her death—once her life-giving medications stopped, life ended. Not immediately. But after her amputation on February 14th, life came crashing down. It was like climbing to the pinnacle of a roller coaster, ever so slowly, clicking over the top . . . and then racing toward the end. Down, up, looping, banking right and smashing left, slowing down to finally reach the end.

Except with all the fear and none of the thrills.

Summary Points

- Hospice means that life is ending, but it doesn't mean life is over. Patients need to keep living and loving. Don't be afraid to start hospice a bit earlier—in many cases it can greatly improve final weeks of life.

- Quality of life matters—a lot. Make care decisions by walking in their shoes, too—not just in your own.

- Hospice care can look a lot like skilled care, but it's definitely different. The focus is comfort, not extending life. That's a monumental shift in thinking.

- Read the contract fine print. Take time to think, pray, and seek wise counsel. Don't simply get the details and sign on the dotted line as if you were buying a used car. Hold hospice staff accountable, and clearly understand what aspects of care are your responsibility. Hospice doesn't provide everything.

Making the decision to enroll Nana into hospice seemed rational at the time. But I had no idea what I was doing (hindsight being 20/20). You will likely consider this option and may need to choose it. Hospice can relieve a good amount of your stress and care burden, though, and frees you to prepare for the inevitable—how best to spend your remaining time together.

Chapter 16

Goodbye Is Just as Hard as You Think

"How lucky I am to have something that makes saying Goodbye so hard."
- Winnie the Pooh

I never had pets growing up. Well, I did have a fish and some parakeets. But no dogs or cats. So, God thought it would be fun to have me marry an animal lover. Someone who prefers big dogs, several at once, and throw in a couple of cats to make it interesting.

Early in our marriage, we had a little Shih Tzu named Snickers. I never genuinely bonded with him. When we put our first house up for sale, we took him to Nana's house to avoid the hassle of dealing with him during realtor showings. We never brought him home, which didn't bother me.

Eventually, I was convinced to try again, and we adopted a miniature schnauzer named Baxter. We got him for free from Craigslist—true story. My requirements to agree to this family addition were minimal: no shedding, no random barking or mess in the house, no chewing my stuff up, and no jumping on the furniture.

Amazingly, Baxter managed to meet all these demands. Over time, he and I came to terms. Our nightly routine included him laying his head on my slipper while I watched TV, worked, or read. This was hilarious since I didn't play with him, barely acknowledged

147

his existence, and only occasionally met any basic needs.

But those eyes. He had the saddest eyes, even when he was deliriously happy. His tail was a nubbin, but the breeder left his ears long. He was darned cute and won me over after several years. I *loved* that dog. I would catch him alone, hold him, and whisper in his floppy ear to keep this our little secret.

About a year ago, he was injured, and during his exam the Veterinarian discovered Baxter had leukemia. We took steps to slow the disease's progress and keep him comfortable, but he knew something was wrong. You could see it in his eyes, reactions, and how he moved. He knew.

After six months, we had no choice but to euthanize him. Monitoring his decline, making that final decision, and watching him die was excruciating. Even though the Vet assured us Baxter would feel no pain and the process would be extremely quick (all true) . . . I'm not sure how to describe my feelings. As a writer, that's tough to admit.

Having Baxter in our family, loving him in life and death, taught me some important lessons.

- Love can come unexpectedly, especially if you don't fight it.
- Dogs truly do love you, no matter what.
- Watching death overtake someone creates such a helpless feeling.
- No amount of preparation or expectation will remove the feeling of surprise when death comes.
- The most loving act is to be there for them at the end.

Death Doesn't Have to Be a Four-Letter Word

Nana had a short "must-have" list related to her death. Make sure she looked good in her coffin. Make sure *no one* ever saw her without her dentures. Play the songs on her list at the funeral. And don't let her die alone—be there with her.

This list was fairly easily accomplished, except for the last item: be there. How would I know when she was close to dying? She had proven to be a tough lady, a master at rebounding. Dementia patients are notorious for having ups and downs, often.

I couldn't be with her 24/7 for days on end. Nana's rehab/hospice facility assured me they knew the signs and would alert me. I trusted them to do what they said. In the end, they didn't teach me or warn me, not days before, or hours before. It's one of my life's biggest regrets, not being with her when she died. She was physically alone. Years later, I sob at times, thinking of her alone.

I don't want you to live with those feelings. Learn to recognize the signs of death. If you work with a strong care facility or hospice program, they'll make sure you have as much forewarning as possible. You see, death comes in stages. Even though each person is different, there is a certain predictability to dying. Having a sense of the order and knowing the signs can help relieve much of the stress of this process. Less stress leads to less fear and fewer regrets.

According to AgingCare, most terminally ill patients will follow the following pattern as they die.[57] Nana followed this almost to a tee, though I didn't recognize it at the time. In each stage, there are steps you can take to maximize your experiences and time together.

- They will have increased drowsiness and generally be less responsive due to slowed metabolism as their body shuts

LIFE GIVING DEMENTIA CARE

down. Visit when they're most alert; even if they can't speak, they can hear you.

- They'll be more restless, confused, agitated, and may have delusions as they lose track of time or forget people. Be calm and reassuring. Don't try to correct them.

- They will withdraw from social interests due to decreased blood flow and oxygen to the brain as their body prepares for death. This might be the time to whisper in their ear that it's alright to *let go*, that you will be fine.

- Appetite and thirst will drop significantly as the body prepares for death and goes into energy conservation mode. Digestion slows and stops. Throw out the rulebook; let them eat or drink whatever and whenever they want. Ice chips, popsicles, Chapstick to keep the lips moist are all good choices.

- They'll likely become incontinent, so adult diapers or even a catheter will become necessary. Keep them clean and comfortable.

- Their skin may become discolored and cool to the touch due to decreased circulation. They may not be cold, though, so use light rather than heavy blankets.

- Breathing will become irregular, and they might make some odd sounds, especially if there are lung issues. All the rattling and shallow breathing is natural and likely not signs of discomfort. Prop them up with a pillow to help them breathe most easily.

- Bright light hurts the eyes. Your instinct will be to make the room bright and cheery, but they might not like that.

- Pain will become more of an issue, so pain meds, soft music, and massage can all help manage any pain. They may seem more disconnected, but they'll still be aware of you.

- They may have involuntary muscle movement, jerks. It doesn't hurt; try not to be startled. Medication may help them sleep better.

I wish I had known these things when Nana was in hospice care. Before her diagnosis, she was always so afraid of dying. Once her dementia took over, I think this fear diminished some. It didn't bother her not knowing what tomorrow held. But I know her fear was still there, was real, and I could have helped her so much more if only I had known what to expect.

It's an Unavoidable Pain, But …

Shel Silverstein authored some of my favorite children's poetry. He saw life and ordinary things through a different lens. His poems illustrated a perspective that, if you adopt it, can lead to greater joy and personal growth along this journey. Your loved one's pain and disease, though devastating, will not last forever. You must cherish your time together.

"Everything in life is transient. Nothing lasts forever. You can't keep things that aren't meant to be kept, but you can enjoy them while they last."
- Shel Silverstein

My daily reality has grown farther and farther from what was my normal. But I hope I still have a sense of humor—help us have a sense of humor. That can help us both weather, and maybe even find joy in, these final days.

"The Snowball" (by Shel Silverstein)[58]

I made myself a snowball
As perfect as can be.
I thought I'd keep it as a pet,
And let it sleep with me.
I made it some pajamas
And a pillow for its head.
Then last night it ran away,
But first—It wet the bed.

This poem cracks me up. Maybe my sharing it seems odd. But here's what I want you to know: life, our time together, is a gift. All of it, even at the end. Just like the snowball in this poem, things will get messy, and we'll deal with some unexpected things. But, with creativity and imagination, you can help us make memories. By this time, I may not be the life of the party, but I'll still be there. Inside, I will hear, and see, and feel.

This is when you may begin to second-guess everything—the decisions made, not made, mistakes, oversights. You may begin to struggle with big-time guilt. These are very natural reactions to what you will experience together. Let me give you permission to feel these emotions; for most people, they are unavoidable.

Being a caregiver is such a courageous act.[59] Loving, and generous. But I've come to believe it is too easy to get in our own way, to be our own worst enemy. We cling to unrealistic self-expectations, trying to be perfect.

Your guilt may flow from the sense you aren't doing enough for them or giving the right care. This only creates more stress. Where are these guilty thoughts coming from?

There will be times you resent your loved one and the living you've lost. The FOMO syndrome—fear of missing out. There will be times you are so tired; you wish it would just end. Now.

If you had any unresolved personal issues with them, those will most certainly bubble to the surface through this illness. It's best to deal with them now, as well as possible under the circumstances, rather than let them fester or, worse yet, be unresolved after their death.

Thanks to our ultra-social, digital culture, you'll have ample opportunity to compare your caregiving, and your loved one's disease, to others dealing with terminal illness. This is unfair. You both are unique and incomparable.

I pray it's not the case, but you may be dealing with your own issues. Problems with your children, spouse, work, health . . . finances.

I see two ways to look at this issue of guilt: you can believe caregiving is *taking* your time and energy, or you can believe you are *giving* your time and energy. Your choice in this will make all the difference in how you emerge from your caregiving experience.

What Is the End Like?

It had been 75 days since Nana entered hospice care. I knew she wasn't doing well, but she was so peaceful and calm. (That should have been a big red flag for me.) They hadn't increased her pain meds, so it never occurred to me that her time was ending. Surely, she would rally yet one more time.

My out-of-state son came home one Sunday afternoon to visit with her, so he, my youngest son, and I drove to her facility. She hadn't eaten or drank much for over a week. Sleep was her norm. We found her curled up in bed, awake but eyes closed. At peace. I lay in bed with her as we talked, holding her hand. Occasionally she would crack a grin, opening her eyes ever so slightly, so we knew she was listening. It was a sunny day, April 17, 2016. After an hour or so, we said so long and how much we loved her. Nana always refused to say goodbye, preferring to say so long—it's far less final.

She mustered enough energy to whisper, eyes closed, "I love you, too." Maybe it sounds a bit theatrical, but I couldn't make this up if I tried. Six hours later I got the call that she had passed.

Why have I stressed for you to avoid guilt? Because I didn't avoid it. I didn't expect it, know how to spot it, or how to reroute the emotional traffic when it came. Why did I leave her that afternoon? I knew she couldn't survive long without food or water. Why did I think that would change, that she would start to eat and drink, that this was a phase, of sorts? Whatever the reason—denial, ignorance, inattention—I missed my chance to be with her at the end. It's my prayer that this book will protect you from the guilt and pain I've felt.

We raced to her facility. Funny, considering she was already gone. I won't describe what I saw. It's just one more scene that would have been so different if someone had been with her. I'll simply say that every fear she had about her death became reality.

Take as much time in the room with them as you need and want. This is important to your healing, to your grieving. There is a process that follows death. It's not especially complicated, but there are many steps involved.

You will need to give staff the funeral home contact (the one you hopefully chose early on). Representatives will arrive to transport the body to the mortuary. Normally, you can choose to be there, or not, while that happens. I stayed, and recommend you do the same if you can. It was comforting to me to see the care they took in moving her, and I think it also helps to hold staff accountable. Ask facility staff when you must clean out the room or return equipment if death occurs at home.

Typically, you'll meet with mortuary staff to complete funeral arrangements (assuming most plans were made prior). Do you catch the point here—make these plans early on? Details like burial vs. cremation, open or closed casket, location of remains, visitation and service times, slide show, service format, communication with the authorities, and friends and family and the public should be fairly simple to navigate if you've done prior planning. That doesn't mean it will be easy. But many people kick into *business mode* until the funeral, and that can help you manage emotions in the short-term.

Remember my comments earlier about being a glass half-full or half-empty person? Your perspective drives every second of your day, just as surely as your brain directs your heart to beat and lungs to breathe. Perspective doesn't command your attention or require instruction. It's just there, affecting all aspects of life. Be sure you keep a positive outlook throughout this journey—that will make this process much more bearable.

Summary Points

- I can't sugar coat it—walking with a loved one as they die will be agonizing. A friend told me her biggest surprise was that, as hard as it was, she learned she could do it. Now more than ever, as we move through the last stage of illness, it's important to relax, flow with your emotions, and make ways to enjoy your time together. Simply love them.

- You need to prepare but understand you may still be surprised when death comes. Then you'll wonder how you could possibly be surprised. Don't go there—your surprise is due to our innate hunger to hope.

- Learn the end-of-life signs so you'll know when to spend more time with your loved one. Whether they can acknowledge you or not . . . they'll know and want you there.

- Try to keep a sense of humor. Seriously (pun intended). Life is fleeting, and we should work to enjoy every second we possibly can.

- Don't second guess yourself and your decisions. You've done your best, and you're loved for that.

They will die. That's basically their job at this point. The quieter they become, the closer death is. Your job is to care for them, to love them, to be loving (there is a difference), and to be present as much as possible. It's not your job to beat yourself up about whether you lived up to your, or anyone else's, ideal. You'll make the absolute best decisions you can when each decision point comes—no more, no less. It's not possible to be fully prepared when they are gone, so don't harbor guilt about your prior thoughts or for feeling surprised. Be at peace with your best effort and give yourself permission to grieve. You've earned it.

Part IV

The After Stage

Chapter 17

Let's Get Down to Business

"Plans are only good intentions unless they immediately degenerate into hard work."
- PETER DRUCKER

Up front disclaimer: I am not an attorney. I am a CPA with a good dose of personal experience, along with several decades of working in business. But the extent of my pure legal knowledge begins and ends with one college business law class.

The school of hard knocks is a tough, but effective, teacher. Through my parents' deaths, I learned some of the more important tasks you should do, and a few things that you shouldn't. So, let's get down to the challenging work of settling the estate.

The Finances

Everyone has an estate at the time of their death. An estate is everything forming their net worth, including all land and real estate, possessions, financial securities, cash, and other assets the individual owns or controls. It can be large, or small; but it's an estate just the same.

First, a quickie law lesson. Probate is the legal process of proving a Last Will and Testament. If a person dies with a will, probate can be simpler, and the executor will have authority to distribute the decedent's assets as directed in their will. If a person dies without a will, they are termed "intestate" and the court, not the family, determines how assets are distributed. Definitely not ideal. If a person has transferred their assets to a trust outside of their will, probate is not involved, and the trust terms rule the day. In my layperson's opinion, a trust is the way to go.

You should carefully review the information in the All About Me folder I suggested in Chapter 7 your loved one create. That will lay the groundwork for what you need to do, and when. The first task to tackle is paying for the funeral. If they made prior plans, and paid for them, this is a non-issue.

But if they made plans and haven't paid, or if they made no plans, payment must be arranged during the funeral planning meeting that happens the day or so after death. This can be done by you or the executor if that's a different person. Most folks will choose one of the following methods.

- Pay with cash or liquid assets, investments, etc.
- Use life insurance proceeds (insurance should already be in place). Obviously, you won't have that cash yet. But give the policy information to the mortuary. They'll confirm coverage and beneficiaries and move forward with planning. Most will do *nothing* until they can confirm that someone has the means to pay in full, lump sum. There generally are no payment plans for funerals, at least not in my experience—they are mostly "cash and bury." Some mortuaries will file the death claims for you. I contacted each of Nana's policy providers directly, myself, to be certain it was handled well. It was simple, companies were extremely kind, and I received the policy proceeds within a few days.
- Use a credit card or get a bank loan.

My father's funeral cost twice as much as Nana's. The day after Nana died, I price shopped caskets online. That's a real thing—Costco even carries them. There don't seem to be many casket manufacturers, only 30–35 in 2020, so the research was straightforward. We bought the identical casket online that we saw at the funeral home for half the cost and had it delivered directly to the mortuary. You do have to act quickly since it takes a few days to ship. Otherwise, you must delay services. But we saved well over $1,500 in 2016. At a minimum, research and pick your mortuary before they die so you don't end up with buyer's remorse from making quick, poorly thought out decisions.

Next up on the to-do list is paying their bills—final medical, debts, home, or care facility costs. If you keep up with this during their illness, things should go smoothly. If they still own their home, or have housing expenses, continue paying those during the estate settlement. No one wants to buy a cold, empty house with no running water, if you get my drift.

Medical bills will trickle in for a few months, so watch for those. You should be able to redirect their mail just by notifying the USPS. Occasionally you may be asked to provide a copy of the death certificate to update accounts (which the mortuary will provide to you—request several copies). Just because you may inherit their assets does not mean you inherit their bills and debts. You do not, and every company I talked with assured me of that fact. Unless laws change, if the estate has sufficient assets to pay the bills after death, you will pay them. If the estate assets are not sufficient, the bills are unpaid and eventually written off by the creditor. You are not required to use life insurance proceeds you receive as beneficiary to pay their debts.

You should check their mail routinely during the illness, keeping track of everyone who will need to be contacted after death. This isn't foolproof. I contacted every single organization that mailed my parents, some multiple times. Years after their death, I still receive mail in their names. Try to contact all of them within the first month, if possible, to let them know of your loved one's passing.

Keep detailed records of assets at the time of death and how every cent is spent or distributed. Include invoices, receipts—all supporting documentation. This is primarily the executor's job, but it can be delegated if the relationships among heirs are strong. Having complete records will help prevent legal action down the road.

The Stuff

My stuff will come in all shapes and sizes. Some things might cause you to scratch your head in wonder—why didn't I sell it, take the money, and run? Or why did I own it at all? There may be some bigger items like a house or cars to handle. Frankly, those are the easy things to handle. It's the stuff inside those big items that might cause you stress. I know you'll honor my stated wished and be a good steward of my estate. But don't lose sleep over this.

You've probably heard the heart wrenching stories of people trying to go through their loved one's stuff in the days, months . . . sometimes years after the funeral. Like most folks who lack first-hand experience, I only understood this to a degree. I knew that sorting through and disposing of clothes, mementos, and such would be depressing, but the person is physically gone, right? Why should it be that hard? There might be several reasons, not all of them emotionally driven.

In the five years since my father's death, I only managed to donate 500 books from his workshop and move a few boxes around. As I write, there are still dozens of records, boxes of clothes, new and old hand and power tools . . . lots of tools . . . collectibles, photography and model building equipment, doo-dads and handy helpers you buy on TV, furniture, and building materials. I'm so afraid I'll toss something important, or valuable, that I'm frozen.

That's the practical reason for being intentional, and extremely careful, as you wade through items. But then there's also the emotional reason.

In the months after his funeral, I didn't do anything with his clothing out of respect for Nana. Plus, I was busy caring for her since I quickly realized my dad had helped her way more than I realized. As her health declined, disposing of his belongings dropped to the bottom of my to-do list.

As a result, his basement workshop is still filled to the rafters. After Nana died, I went through their closet and dressers to donate most items. Since they sold their home and lived with my family, that's all they owned besides two cars. I'll be honest—the process of touching, of folding and bagging everything, was both agonizing and joyous. Every item seemed to have some memory attached to it. The lingering scent of my dad's Old Spice and Nana's White Shoulders cologne. Stains from Nana's many spills that we didn't catch before washing. (By the way, Dreft, the baby detergent, works great on old food stains.) All of her left foot shoes, orphaned after her amputation, and the times we laughed until we cried at the absurd number of shoes she had, mostly black. Ties we gifted to my dad and remembering he would wear several at once just to be goofy and honor the gifts. The t-shirts he'd buy on his semi-annual trips delivering snowbirds' cars back and forth between Chicago and Florida. T-shirts he never wore.

I knew my parents very well. The fact they didn't leave me any specific instructions about their stuff was honestly not an issue. I knew which items were important, to check between book pages or in unlikely spots for money or collectibles, and what trinkets were bought on a whim and of no lingering value.

I don't want you to have to guess. I'll leave you The List. Whether you ultimately decide to keep certain items, or not, at least you'll know the story behind them to make a semi-informed decision. I want you to know why an item made The List. And if it's super-duper important, its disposition will be in my will. In the end, I have no say in the matter. After my estate is settled, you'll do what you want with your inherited stuff. I wouldn't want to take any of it with me, even if I could. What good would it be to me?

The Egyptian Pharaohs were buried with everything they thought the deceased might need in the afterlife, since they believed in "little g" gods. When the tombs were opened millennia later, their remains and their stuff still sat there. I once read about a guy who was so worried about what his relatives would do with his stuff that he arranged to be buried inside his antique Cadillac. He had to buy multiple burial plots to accommodate it. Such a waste.

That's not me, or most folks. I'm a collector of things that have a memory, some emotion attached. Nothing terribly big. Maybe you are the same. Baseball cards because I had 26 boy cousins and didn't want to be bored on my visits. All kinds of Disney plates, pins, books, and figurines because I love Disney, had a mom who bought me anything I wanted, and have visited often to celebrate milestone events. I have artwork and ceramics my kids made or bought on family trips to Colorado, Outer Banks, Marco Island, or Europe. Hallmark ornaments . . . too many, but at least our tree wasn't bare as the kids left home and took their ornament dowry along.

If something makes it into my will or on The List, I see value in it, and I hope you will, too. Most people will have a "wish list" related to their death if they take the time to think about it. You should always ask them. I have a brief list of "pleases." Please respect my stated wishes. Please don't fight with others over my stuff. Please don't just swoop in, box it all up, and send it away on a 1-800-I-Got-Junk truck without thought.

I know the stuff, the assets, and bills are just things; processes to finish, roads to take, things that might spark a memory. But the stuff isn't your loved one—they'll be gone. Just like every other part of this journey, though, stuff offers opportunities to laugh, and to grow—to begin healing.

Summary Points

- Settling the estate is hard work, but your prior planning will pay off. Don't be afraid, and take your time.

- Work the plan, don't be pressured, and get trusted help when needed to settle financial matters.

- Please honor requests made in their will. And don't just toss it—there's probably value there. You might as well sell things and use the proceeds for yourself or to donate.

It takes an average of six to nine months to settle an estate.[60] You'll be surprised at how long it may take for bills to arrive. During this process, you'll still be focused on finishing everything well. But when this is done, you need to focus 100% on healing; healing physically and emotionally from your extended stint as a caregiver. Healing your relationships as needed. And learning how to miss your loved one in a healthy way.

Chapter 18

Healing Is Not for the Faint of Heart

*"A broken heart heals when we allow the healing
to go as deep as the wound went."*
- BETH MOORE

Our bodies are intentionally designed to manage multiple functions without requiring thought or action on our part. A beating heart. Breathing. Digestion and sweating, to name just a few. Vital life processes that sustain us. Healing is like this.

You've probably had this happen ... you have an itch, so you reach to scratch. What do you find but a scab? You don't know when you got that cut, or how, but your body has already taken over to protect and heal. In fact, it itches because most of the healing is done.

Science tells us the biological process of healing involves numerous steps, a complex cascade of events. Of course, we know that the deeper the wound, the greater the body's need for healing. Sometimes the body needs a little help, sometimes a lot. Those helpful bandages, stitches, or antibiotics all coordinate to boost what our body is already doing on its own. Big hurts will only heal well with care and intentionality. If we pay minimal attention, they may still heal, but poorly. Scars or continued pain can result.

If we ignore them, big wounds may never heal, or the scars will be worse than the wound. If those big wounds are emotional, what kind of Band-Aid can help?

One Is the Loneliest Number

You can't heal alone; not well, anyway. We're created as social beings who crave community. Other people are the emotional Band-Aid you'll need. I'm not talking about having a party and pretending the pain will simply disappear. You can find groups or tools to fit your personality and unique needs, if you look.

Take CaringBridge, for example. CaringBridge connects people during a health crisis.[61] They join patients and their tribe with the broader community of folks who want to help, who want updates—people who love you and care, so no one feels alone in this journey.

This site doesn't just provide an outlet for caregivers to pour out their heart. Through the stories people share, it inspires. Friends, neighbors, and co-workers checking in for a patient's update get to experience, first-hand, the courage, struggles, hope, and growth of patients and caregivers alike.

I found a page on their website titled, "19 Inspirational Quotes About Hope and Healing."[62] Some were especially inspiring and help illustrate what I believe is your best perspective.

"Barn's burnt down—Now I can see the moon."
- Haiku Poem by Mizuta Masahide

"Life isn't about waiting for the storm to pass ... It's about learning to dance in the rain." - Vivian Greene

"The sun never quits shining. Sometimes, clouds just get in the way."
- Unknown

"Most folks are as happy as they make up their minds to be."
- Abraham Lincoln

"Change is inevitable. Growth is optional." - John Maxwell

Remember, I'm a glass half-full gal. You need to appreciate, and ponder, the truths and perspectives within each of these thoughts. Do you see the common thread?

Positivity Leads to Growth . . .
Growth Leads to Healing

Each quote illustrates that the bigger picture overflows with hope, whether or not you can initially see it. Surrounding this knowledge is the firm belief that, to see this picture, you must *set your mind*. It's a decision made, sometimes weekly or daily, sometimes minute by minute. But regardless of timing, this decision must be made. The more challenging your circumstances, the more intentional is your decision to seek hope.

Does it seem odd to talk about hope when you are in the midst of grief? Not actually.

Throughout these pages, I've advocated for growth. Yours and your loved one's. This was my experience, growth through my caregiving, and there's research to support this outcome.

In my caregiver research, I noticed that most information and help available focuses on caregiver survival, or coping—on the challenges you'll encounter. There's not much talk about the upside of this journey.

But, studies have shown that a majority, even as high as 90%, of caregivers experience personal growth.[63] Especially if the primary caregiver is an adult child of the patient. How is this growth defined?

In phrases like: learning to prioritize better and evaluate what is truly important in life; having all that extra time with your loved one; becoming a more caring, compassionate person; enjoying improved health due to a slower lifestyle. Caregivers reported building stronger, and more, community connections, and learning to reframe one's circumstances and lean into one's faith. And there were more.

We know growth comes from challenge, from being pushed. That doesn't stop me from rolling my eyes when athletes say, "No pain, no gain," on the way to six-pack abs. But it's true. Sometimes we only have a vague, foggy vision of the path between the journey's beginning and end. We need to keep faith in the process and outcome, even if we're not exactly sure of the steps in between.

We need to be comfortable with that unknown part.

"Life is like a camera. Just focus on what's important and capture the good times. Develop from the negatives, and if things don't work out, just take another shot." - Ziad K. Abdelnour

My dad was an amateur photographer and built a darkroom in our basement. Think of this analogy. Back in the day, when cameras were used instead of phones for photography, folks put film in a camera, pointed it at a person or object, and clicked a button, not knowing if the picture was any good. To find out, they took the film to a lab for development. That process took place in a "darkroom," where a combination of darkness and chemicals transformed the film into pictures.

The caregiver journey is a lot like that. Only by going through the darkness, through the pain of transformation, can you see the end result—a clearly developed picture—growth.

A Grief Timeout

My college Psychology 101 course taught me the Kübler-Ross five stages of grief: shock and denial, anger, bargaining, depression, and finally, acceptance.[64] You'll move through all of them. How long it takes, and the fallout from each, will be different for every person and will largely depend on your determination to move forward—the daily choice for hope.

Psychology 101 did *not* teach me there are also several different types of grief.[65] I learned through my own research and experience. Caregivers who help loved ones with chronic illness, particularly those involving cognitive decline like dementia, often experience grief not only after their person dies, but all along the journey prior to death. Sometimes the grief can seem almost constant.

No wonder caregivers seem to have such a high rate of personal illness.

Our grief will often come from the nearly unending, unacceptable changes that I'll experience. I'll move from being Mom as you knew me, to being Mom who needs help getting from point A to point B; Mom who can't pick her clothes out or put them on. I'll become Mom who needs help to eat, and Mom who doesn't remember your name . . . or recognize you at all. As each shift happens, grief is a natural emotion—for you, and for me. As long as I'm able, let's share this process, supporting each other.

And what about grief from your own losses? Your loss of freedom, of control in life. Possibly loss of relationships, peace, or financial security. The loss of the future you had planned—either the kind of future, or the timing.

Caregivers have so much to tackle and manage that it's easy to push forward and ignore all the caution signs. Build some railroad crossings into your life so you will pause, stop, and evaluate. Look both ways and wait. Your healing depends on this.

As your loved one slips away from being the person you've known, you might experience *Anticipatory Grief.* With every step backward, you may mourn the loss of who they were. This can go on for a long time, and it'll hurt a great deal. Some might say this process is more painful than their actual death.

I busied myself with the daily work of caregiving for Nana. I knew she was changing, but I didn't accept what was happening. Denial, most would say. I didn't see that I was losing her—only that, for the first time in my life, my mom was allowing me to truly help her. She was relying on me. This was an unexpected, and amazing, feeling at the time.

Anticipatory Grief hit me through my guilt, not my mourning. I was so tired, so frustrated, and deeply discouraged watching her dementia take over. When I could no longer ignore her changes, at times I wished she would die sooner than later. The woman I knew would not want to live like she was—not in a million years. Nana was not fully aware of her decline, living in blissful ignorance for the most part. I was the one struggling to balance my memories of who she once was with the constant demands of caregiving. I found myself wishing the present circumstances would end.

Even though these are very normal reactions, years later, I still hold deep guilt for having those thoughts, and I'm still working through that part of my healing.

The upside of my guilt was, you got it—growth. I became more patient. Things no longer had to be perfect, or close to it. Okay was often . . . well . . . good enough. I stopped seeing my mom as defective and sick. Instead I saw her as she was—changing, but still my mom. Not forgetting, or spilling, or being slow on purpose just to irritate me. She was doing her best, and I learned to do mine.

The next grief type: *Ambiguous Loss.* We experience this when it feels like the patient is there, but in truth isn't. This is an especially strong type of grief when dealing with cognitive illnesses like dementia, stroke, or a traumatic brain injury.

As a caregiver, you experience wild emotional swings when your loved one's behavior or personality takes a dive, then seems to fully reverse course. If they can do that once, why can't they do it whenever?

This tendency toward super quick changes in lucidity was illustrated so well in *The Notebook.*[66] One minute during a visit, Noah is clearly a complete stranger to his wife, Ally. But then instantly, for a moment, it's like the lights were turned on, and she recognizes him as her beloved Noah. They have this very brief, tender moment together, which just as suddenly ends with Ally jerking away, screaming for help to stop this stranger from touching her.

This emotional rollercoaster can become all too routine and be maddening if you don't expect it and prepare. I never managed to overcome my surprise when this happened with Nana. But I learned not to take it personally. That was real growth for me.

In the end, as with most dementia caregivers, I experienced the grief of death. It's intense, painful, and lasts a lot longer than you expect. Grief is a very normal emotional response—you are experiencing a great loss. They won't physically be there to listen to (and not get) your jokes, comfort you when things go wonky, or laugh or cry at the same movie scenes for the 100th time.

There will be a void. You can be intentional and fill it with love and memories; or you can try to ignore it and let negativity creep in to fill it for you. Either way, the void will be filled. That's where healing comes in.

Tears: Band-Aids for the Heart

Grief affects every part of you—social, emotional, physical, and spiritual. Maybe you'll let others see your grief, and maybe not. I do know that there is a time and place to "let it out." But if you shove it all down, keep it inside, indefinitely, you're only hurting yourself.

Harry Potter was healed by tears in the second franchise film, *Harry Potter and the Chamber of Secrets.*[67] The Basilisk, a giant snake living in the chamber, wounded Harry. As Harry's life hangs in the balance, a mythical Phoenix named Fawkes swoops in to gently drop tears on his injured arm. Magically, the wound heals. Phoenix tears, it seems, have healing powers. I believe there's healing through our tears, too.

There's a fair amount of research available about why we cry and how crying, or not, affects us. It's true that women cry more than men, in general—an average of around forty-seven times a year for gals and seven for guys.[68] Cultural views may be a big part of the difference, but that has been changing. Historically, a crying man was seen as weak. In recent years, this has flipped completely. Now, strong men are expected to cry, and the weak keep it all inside. Tears are a badge of courage and symbol of confidence and caring.

Researchers have learned that tears caused by varying stimuli have different chemical content. Emotional tears hold toxins built up from stress and pain.[69] Our bodies need to get rid of that stuff to feel better. Apparently nine out of ten criers feel better after their sob fest. [70] Maybe that's why women outlive men—we cry more.

Here's a fun fact: The Japanese believe so strongly in the health benefits of crying that it's become a business.[71] You can go to crying clubs, interact with sad or emotional movies or songs, and cry to your heart's content . . . for a fee. They even offer classes in how to cry better.

I'm not saying that tears are a "magic pill" to instantly heal your grief. I am saying that it's important to connect with your feelings and not ignore them. There are many ways to do this.

Healing 101

I'm a fan of the J.K. Rowling series, *Harry Potter*, so let's look at another analogy taken from those films. In the sixth and eight movies, we encounter a magical dish called a Pensieve and a cabinet filled with glass vials of tears.[72] Empty a vial into the dish, and you are able to relive the memories contained within the tears. Not quite as simple as watching a digital video, but it works. As he's dying, Harry's teacher, Severus Snape, orders Harry to "save them [his tears]." Using the Pensieve and the tears, Harry experiences Snape's most significant memories. By sharing his memories, Snape helped Harry to heal years of pain, correct several destructive beliefs, and pave the way for Harry's future. Memories hold power.

Memories can be attached to events, places, music, people, things. Some things we value aren't just objects, but rather a tool to get past grief and pain. Photos and videos of my parents, especially of Nana and my dad in their last year, mean so much to me and have been part of my path to healing.

About a year before my dad died, I bought a stuffed bear and a bunny that could record a voice message. I intended to have each of my parents record a short message to me. After they were gone, I would be able to squeeze a paw and hear my mom or dad's voice expressing their love for me, telling a joke . . . whatever they recorded.

I didn't ask my dad to record a message in the bear before his death. In fact, it's still in a box on my bedroom chair. But I did record Nana in the bunny, and that's one of my most precious possessions.

She was fairly deep into her dementia when we recorded, so her first words were, "I don't know what to say [giggle, giggle]." Every day she'd tell me I was the "light of her life." So, the power of repetition kicked in, and those were the next words she recorded, adding that she loved me and then laughing.

I squeeze the bunny every few days even now, years later. It's a tremendous comfort to me. I would highly recommend you find some way to record your loved one sharing their thoughts and feelings about you. This is exactly why I bought a copy of my sons' favorite childhood books, recorded myself reading them, and gave them the DVD and books one Christmas. I'm quite emotional and cry easily, so recording myself reading them was tough—it took several attempts. But they'll always have that piece of our history, our relationship; a handy reminder of how much I love them. Connecting to memories of your loved one will be important for your healing.

Healing Steps, Healing Hearts

Is healing truly as simple as just crying, a lot? No, but that's a great start. The true foundation of your healing is the grieving process itself. Be sure to move through all 5 stages, completely. There are differing opinions on how many stages exist. Some experts say it's 10, others 12.[73]

The point is that healing is personal; your experience will probably be different than mine. In general, it's natural to experience some level of denial. Your faith may be shaken—faith in yourself, others, the future, institutions . . . maybe even in God. Regardless of which stages you experience, resolving your grief will involve acceptance—discovering a renewed faith in life, joy, and a sense of peace.

Let's talk about steps toward healing you can take after your caregiver days.

- Express your feelings and let it out. Remember the benefits of crying.
- Join a support group or connect with friends and relatives who can relate, maybe have been there and done that.
- Delay major decisions for a year, in general. It's tough to think clearly, and if you inherit much, you don't want to regret choices made during this time.
- Expect to need at least a full year to work through your emotions. All of those "firsts" after their death. The first Christmas or birthday without gifts. The first Memorial Day, Labor Day, or July 4th without those special baked beans. The first time you see a Disney commercial and remember how much they loved the mouse. It'll be difficult, and emotion may hit unexpectedly. It will help to know this will happen.
- Please take care of yourself. When my maternal grandfather died, Nana shut down for nearly three months. She couldn't function. My dad eventually gave her a good talking to, and she began to accept her loss. Don't let that happen to you. Eat well even if you don't feel like it. Rest and exercise. Get whatever professional help you need. There's no shame in asking. Lean on others and your faith, not on artificial support.
- Take time to remember your loved one—don't run and hide. Life is for the living, and they would want you to enjoy life. They'll always be part of you, and your memories can be comforting. It might hurt at first, but remember them on their birthday, and yours, on Mother's or Father's Day and

other key dates. Once you move beyond the daily challenges of caregiving, you may see life and that relationship with new clarity—your experiences, and how you have grown through this journey. Since Nana passed, my appreciation for her has grown tremendously. I love being reminded of her likes and dislikes, of what made her laugh and what made her mad. It's like looking through a window to see not only who she was, but who I am because of her, and that always warms my heart.

Healing doesn't mean forgetting. Pain always leaves a scar to remind us of lessons learned . . . if we let it. For some, it might remind them of the pain, for others, the loss. But I pray your scar is a badge of courage, a reminder of the road you traveled with your loved one in sadness and joy, in struggles and laughter. It's like swimming upstream against the current, fighting slowly toward the shore. Only by looking back do you realize just how far you've come. To heal, you must decide that your caregiving time has a purpose— to love along the journey into their final days, and through this experience, to grow into your very best self.

"The flower that blooms in adversity is the rarest and most beautiful of all."
- Walt Disney

Epilogue

Who Cared for Whom?

"Rivers know this: there is no hurry. We shall get there someday."
- Winnie the Pooh

My family was fortunate—my mother may not have recognized anyone outside of family, but she died knowing exactly who we were, with the ability to communicate with us even in her extreme weakness. We didn't face blank stares, total confusion, or fear in Nana's eyes, thinking we were strangers.

For those who do reach this point in their loved one's illness, my encouragement to search for and find a little ray of sunshine each day may ring hollow. Please understand that I don't mean to diminish the deep pain and anguish caregivers experience when their loved one's mind is completely absent.

Everyone who deals with terminal illness is unique; so is every caregiver, and every caregiving experience. Through my caregiving, and that of so many others I've known, I am convinced it's possible to experience daily peace and joy on this journey, even on the darkest days.

For 18 chapters, we've discussed how to provide loving care for someone through dementia or terminal illness; I've shared my caregiving experience and lessons I learned along the way.

I've come to believe, though, that I received far more care from my "care-ees" than I gave.

You can spend energy and emotion being angry about how your loved one changed, how they are not the mom or dad that you knew and loved. Or you can celebrate who they have become. I've wondered . . . maybe the "dementia Nana" was who she truly was, inside, all along. But life, circumstances, and pain buried her true self, so no one could see it, not even Nana.

I don't know for sure. What I do know is that so much of what I learned during my time as her caregiver was due to Nana and her dementia changes.

- I learned to laugh at the ridiculousness of things that happen to our bodies.
- I learned to sit, to just be with someone, not doing a darned thing except enjoying their company.
- I learned what real courage looks like, watching my mom accept her new normal, over and over, as it changed.
- I learned it is possible to put even the most intense pride aside so you can move forward, to simply enjoy today.
- I learned how to care for an adult in a whole new way. It's definitely not the same as caring for a child . . . but I'll be honest—there are similarities.
- I became more organized. You know, the whole "necessity is the mother of invention" thing.
- I learned that pursuing perfection isn't a goal as much as it is a distraction.
- I learned to be more comfortable around sick and dying people.
- I learned that there are many, many ways to communicate love and respect. We don't need words, or hours. A soft touch, a warm embrace, or a gentle smile will do the trick.

I never planned to have "dementia caregiver" on my resumé. Caregiving was incredibly difficult, and at times, I wanted to run away. But in the end, the experience had a profound impact on my growth as a person, mother, friend, and wife. Maybe some caregivers describe their experience in terms like "painful," "exhausting," "endless." These feelings are real, but they don't have to define you or your journey. Planning, a clear view of reality, and an uplifting, positive attitude mixed with daily optimism can make all the difference.

For me, caring for my parents, especially my mom through her disease, was . . . life giving.

Appendix

Caregiver Family Interviews

Being a caregiver can be a very solitary, isolating experience. No matter how hard the people around you may try, no one can truly understand what you are living through unless they've walked in your shoes.

At the same time, those closest to you—your spouse, children, siblings—have their own unique experience as they watch and hopefully support you during your time as a caregiver. This experience changes everyone in your circle, and especially those you love. They see the effect on you as a caregiver, on your relationship with them and others, and on their relationship with each other.

Everyone most closely involved will be changed, forever. I can say with all confidence, though, that you have a good deal of control on this outcome. As I've shared throughout this book, attitude, patience, humility, love, and respect will win the day.

It never occurred to me to necessarily seek out support during my mother's illness. I rarely talked with others about my struggles outside of immediate family. In hindsight, I wish I had. Several years after my mother passed, I wanted to know what others in my circle saw and experienced during her dementia; what friends who were caregivers experienced with their loved one.

To gather their thoughts, I developed a simple survey for each to answer about their caregiving experience. This included my husband and sons. Reading each person's thoughts caused me to have unexpected feelings. Excruciatingly painful, yet completely freeing.

As I relived the experience through their eyes, I realized that I have grieved losing my mother, but I'd never grieved losing that time in my life, losing that part of me. I haven't sobbed that much since my mother's funeral.

In this appendix, I share their unedited comments, observations, and advice for you as a caregiver. Each person's interview is preceded by a little background about their caregiving role. Their responses are written in first person, from their perspective. It's our prayer that in sharing their insight as those who have "been there and done that", you will gain a sense of peace and build confidence as you travel this caregiver road.

AMY:

Amy's mother was diagnosed with cancer at 84 and fought the disease for eighteen months before her death in 2020. Amy, her siblings, and immediate family provided care during her mom's final two months, with the assistance of friends and eventually in-home contracted help.

QUESTIONS & RESPONSES:

What was your biggest surprise in caring for your loved one?

The biggest surprise was that we can do the hard things, and for us, one of those hard things was caring for her most personal needs. In the end, it became a very holy and precious gift to care for her in this way. The first year of her illness involved taking her to normal medical visits, a few trips to the ER, some hospitalizations, scheduling appointments, purchasing her groceries, etc. We thought that was hard because it was disruptive to the lives we were living. But the last two months of her life, when things quickly changed and

24/7 care was suddenly needed, we lived a whole new level of "hard." Mom was always very capable and active, even as her disease progressed. She accepted our help, but she would say, "Dear heavens, I'm so sorry you have to do this." We assured her that we were so happy to be there to help her, and that it really was ok. Bless her heart, she was often mortified at having her children and grandchildren have to clean up after she soiled herself or her bedding. I often thought to myself that I couldn't believe I was doing these things. It was not fun. It was hard and uncomfortable and messy. But then I'd look at her precious face and the love she felt as we cared for these most intimate things (and the sadness in her eyes knowing she needed help) and I knew this was a holy moment. I'm not saying any of this was comfortable, but it wasn't hard to do in the end. It felt like such an act of love and service; we were so happy to be able to help her.

What was the best decision you made, and why?

Getting help, and receiving help immediately when we were told she needed 24/7 care. We didn't delay. We figured the time would come, so we had already been looking at home health care services. That was so smart, because her condition changed literally within 24 hours, and since we had already been looking we were able to have help within a few days. It's a good idea to line up several organizations in case your first choice is not available. It took us contacting three in-home, long term care groups to get to one with availability when we had the need. If we had to take time to research when the need arose, we would have been rushed, mom's care would have suffered, and we might have made a poor decision.

Another thing is we set up a google sheet as a daily help calendar with a 24 hour schedule of caregivers. While I was the primary one to ensure the slots were filled, my entire family had access to the sheet and could add their names to the empty time slots. I had a long talk with my (all adult) kids and husband, and we agreed we would care for her together as a family. No one would be asked to do more than they could, and no one would fuss about how much or little someone else did. I set the ground rules, and thankfully, everyone was gracious to each other. We continued to increase her day/night care as needed. I did draw a line that I would not spend the night with her. Instead, we added a night shift from home health care. That was a gift to me, and thankfully, mom had a policy to cover a portion of the cost. As primary caregiver, I had to allow the load to be shared or I would have fallen completely apart. I had to trust those who stepped in to help. It's critical to be understanding and supportive. I was so tired, but I knew I had people who would help carry the burden.

I found a wonderful online site that allowed friends and neighbors to sign up for a variety of daytime needs (https://www.giveinkind.com) from stopping by for lunch, taking mom to appointments, or giving me a much needed break from caregiving. We built a village of wonderful helpers!

What was your biggest mistake, and how did you overcome it (or did you)?

As I mentioned, we worked with a home health care company, and also with a woman who operated her own private home health care service. We were more lax with her as she was also a friend of my mom's, in terms of obtaining daily or weekly documentation of care. Later, when we applied for reimbursement from her long term care policy, we were denied because we couldn't get documentation/confirmation of the work she'd done. That was a mistake, as well as not knowing exactly what the long term care policy provider required when filing for benefit reimbursement.

What is the most important thing a new caregiver should know or remember?

It's hard. You can do hard things, but you will need help. And that in-home hospice care (IHHC) isn't what you think it is. Our reality did not meet the IHHC brochure or intake description. I wish I could write a blog or book about IHHC, because no one talks about it. In the end, we got much of what we needed, but it was a battle. On the day of mom's death, the hospice nurse questioned our request for her to be with us, and as a result we weren't prepared for how quickly mom would decline. I still need to write a tell-all letter to the hospice director...and we continue to process the entire IHHC experience months later.

Did you grow as a person through this experience, and if so, how?

Yes. I learned to always be honest about how you feel. Caregiving is so hard, and so exhausting, but, of course I'd choose to do it all again. God provided us with the strength and perspective to do what was needed. It's critical to be transparent so others can know when and how to step in and help, but then you must let them! People want to help, and I quickly learned I couldn't do it all. The entire experience has caused me to reexamine my priorities, particularly the number of hours I work. I am still allowing that to impact me. There was great joy in caring for my mom, but it was really hard, so we purposefully CHOSE to find or create joy. We laughed a lot, teased a lot, spent lots of time with her. We learned to give each other space and loved each other well as a family. Everyone shared the load and understood our purpose as a family. It was beautiful. My mom saw it and felt the love. I have no idea why God gave us that gift. We were not necessarily expecting that, but she, and all of us, received it, and we are all still so grateful for that time together with her and as a family. I look back and can say with absolute certainty that we walked through that terrible time with joy and love and very few regrets. It continues to impact how I approach each day.

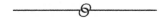

LINDA:

Linda's father, Bob, developed dementia in his late eighties. Along with her sister and brother, Linda cared for her dad until his death at age ninety-two. Bob spent this time living at his home, in an assisted-living facility, and finally with his son's family.

QUESTIONS & RESPONSES:

What was your biggest surprise in caring for your loved one?

The loved one that I cared for was Bob, which was my dad. He lived to be 92 years old. In the last few years of his life, he developed dementia. For a while, my dad lived in his own house. My sister and I would buy his groceries, pay his bills, assist with cooking meals, and take him to doctor appointments. It was too much for us to keep up with since we both worked full-time jobs besides caring for Dad. Dad also developed a condition where he could not swallow his food and had to be fed with a G-tube. My sister and I would administer some of the G-tube feedings, and we hired caregivers to do other feedings while we were at work. Later, my dad fell and needed more assistance. So, he stayed at an assisted living facility for a while. My biggest surprise in caring for dad was how much he changed in only one week. When we would come visit, we'd point out family members in photos, and he didn't know who they were. We would review the photos and tell stories to jog his memory, which would create a spark for him to begin to remember. But his memory was short-lived, it seemed to fade as soon as we left. The next time we would come for a visit, we would start all over again. The most difficult time was his last couple of months of his life, when he developed other health issues, and even forgot who my sister and I were. That was heart wrenching. It was the greatest joy when something sparked his memory, and he knew us again!

What was the best decision you made, and why?

My dad stayed in an assisted living facility for a while after he fell at his house, and he needed medical assistance with his G-tube feedings. Because he had the G-tube, he had to be in the nursing care area of the facility. The facility was understaffed, so the only time anyone interacted with Dad was when they did his G-tube feedings. My sister and I would visit Dad every evening after work, and he had been left laying asleep all day in bed. My sister, brother, and I discussed other options. My brother offered to take Dad to live with him and his wife at their house. They have a large house, although an hour away for my sister and I to visit. But, we felt it was the best option. My sister-in-law helped with Dad, since she stayed home all day. But, we also paid caregivers to care for dad during the weekdays. My sister and I would visit every Saturday and spend the day with Dad at my brother's house. The best decision that we made was having Dad live at my brother's house rather than the assisted living facility. Since the facility was understaffed, Dad would get up to go the restroom and forget to use his walker. He fell a few times, one time resulting in a hospital visit because he fell and hit his head on the floor. Also, at the facility, he laid in bed all day, and his dementia got worse, because no one interacted with him, besides the times my sister and I visited. I believe Dad lived longer and had a better quality of life while staying at my brother's house.

What was your biggest mistake, and how did you overcome it (or did you)?

During the last few months of Dad's life, he was in hospice at my brother's house. Dad would get out of bed and seemed confused, saying he had to go somewhere, but wasn't sure where. The hospice nurse recommended giving Dad antipsychotic drugs to calm him, but it seemed to get him more agitated. I believe our biggest mistake was agreeing to give Dad those drugs at the end of his life. The drugs made Dad more confused, disoriented, weak, and unsteady on his feet. He fell a few times. His end of life came soon after that.

What is the most important thing a new caregiver should know or remember?

The most important thing that a new caregiver should know is not to blame yourself for whatever happens. Do your personal best to give your loved one the care they need, but you are not in control of the outcome.

It's easy to tell yourself, "if only" I had done this or that. Your loved one is in God's hands, and there is only so much you can do. Be sure to take care of yourself! You must get breaks and help from others, so you have something left to give.

Did you grow as a person through this experience, and if so, how?

Yes, I grew tremendously as a person. I found inner strength that I didn't know existed in me. I also grew in my faith, knowing that God was in control all along.

———————⊙———————

J.K.:

J.K. and his brother provided care for their mother, Maxine, during her dementia. Being a widow, Maxine selected a residential facility early on that could allow her to transition from independent living to increasing care levels. Before her dementia, she was a vibrant woman, well known and very active in her community (which has a rich, 150-year history). Maxine was the official township historian.

QUESTIONS & RESPONSES:

What was your biggest surprise in caring for your loved one?

The cognitive impact of the disease caught us off guard. For example, we could talk to mom on the phone early after the diagnosis, but after about 10 minutes of visiting she said she couldn't hear us anymore. We realized that the brain tired after talking for a while and stopped processing her hearing. The same was true in our visits with her—she would tire and could not process information after that point.

What was the best decision you made, and why?

Mom had chosen the facility for her care and we concurred. It proved to be a wonderful choice because the facility had a large open room with the rooms for patients around the outside. That made it very easy for mom to come and go from the common area without needing to find her room down a hallway.

What was your biggest mistake, and how did you overcome it (or did you)?

Mom was living independently early in the process and there was no facility based assisted living. It was several months into a deteriorating situation before we realized how serious mom's failures were becoming. Even visiting aid was a problem because they did not track with how mom was fooling them in her performance or her willingness to cooperate in areas like taking meds. We were busy, with children still at home, and not checking on her daily. Our frustrations were increasing, and we had to learn from experience because the doctor and others were not coaching us. We still look back at this period with sadness, wishing we had understood more at the time.

What is the most important thing a new caregiver should know or remember?

While dementia impacts people in different ways, there are patterns to how deterioration takes place. Memory loss also affects cognitive processing in ways we did not know. The challenge comes in the unpredictability of the rate and steps of deterioration. This is compounded by the tiring effect of ongoing problems that cannot be fixed. Communication with onsite caregivers is never perfect and very dependent on their time, but that should not be allowed to govern how the family is informed and a plan for care kept in place. We wish we had sought out good coaching beyond the doctors and the facility staff as support for coping with the difficulties we faced.

Did you grow as a person through this experience, and if so, how?

Hardship is a difficult teacher, and the lessons are often learned after the fact when there is no chance to recoup the time. We learned the disappointment and frustration of dementia the hard way. In the midst of that we also learned to treasure the moments when mom came out of her shell to be herself for just a moment. It pleased us that she also enjoyed the funny moments and could laugh with us. We are not specialists, but we are more compassionate and understanding than before this period of life began. We hope we are more prepared if we should ever face this again.

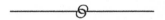

SUSAN:

Susan and her siblings worked together to care for their mother, Carrie, for several years during her struggle with dementia. Carrie lived in a skilled care facility, but before diagnosis she was an elementary school music teacher for 20 years. Active in her community and church, she most enjoyed time with her children, 14 grandchildren and 15 great-grandchildren.

QUESTIONS & RESPONSES:

What was your biggest surprise in caring for your loved one?

How she retained her ability to switch on maternal instinct and advice when around great-grandchildren. To the end she was able to share interesting and valuable tidbits of parenting knowledge.

What was the best decision you made, and why?

Thinking in terms of quality of life for my mom vs. quantity of life. Making each day with her the best for her possible. Living in the moment with each visit.

What was your biggest mistake, and how did you overcome it?

Not realizing early on that something was amiss. Thinking she was always mad at me because she was defensive and argumentative when I challenged her about things she said but didn't recall.

Unnecessary tension that was instantly gone once I realized it was dementia and short-term memory loss, not animosity.

What is the most important thing a new caregiver should know or remember?

Don't argue - ever. Just lead the discussion to a new topic and keep things light. Learn the art of redirection.

Did you grow as a person through this experience, and if so, how?

I think I became more patient? I do know I aged during the process, probably recognizing for the first time my own future growing old.

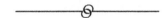

ADAM:

Adam is our eldest son and was out of our home and married by the time of mom's diagnosis. I called him the "golden grandchild" because he was the first on both sides of our family. During mom's illness, he lived nearby and visited regularly. All our sons are observers, and intelligent; little gets past them. Adam is especially so. We used to move little things around the house to see if he noticed. He always did, even as a toddler. He was especially kind during this journey.

QUESTIONS & RESPONSES:

What was it like to watch Nana change during her dementia?

Beyond being sad and scary and all that, it was difficult to continue thinking of her as the same person. Obviously she had changed and was continuing to change and wasn't the same in the sense that she was forgetting who she was, who she'd been, and who we were, but she was still Lois; she was still who she'd always been even if she didn't remember it. But it was difficult to think of her that way when she was so different and didn't remember so much. She never did seem to completely forget who I was though so that helped some. It was scary to see it progressing and know it could happen to other people in our family in the future.

What do you think were the biggest impacts on me as her primary caregiver?

The stress, all the time you had to spend taking care of her and dealing with the things that popped up, making sure she didn't do anything to hurt herself when she still lived at home then making sure she was properly cared for when she lived in the nursing facility. Having to see the changes in her daily and having to deal with her acting differently than she normally would and mainly directing that toward you.

How did this affect my relationship with you, short and long term?

I don't think it had much of an impact on our relationship in that it changed anything or shifted the dynamic or the way I viewed you. The biggest impact was just talking about it and hearing what it was like from you and/or being able to infer what it was like.

How did this experience impact you personally, both positive and negative?

The obvious negative impact is it's very hard/difficult/sad to see that happening to someone and that's part of my memory of her. Positive—I feel it helped me be able to talk with and interact with older people, I can recognize when someone has dementia or likely has it or some form of it and I can communicate with them. It also has helped me relate to and talk with family members and caretakers of people w/dementia.

What is your best advice to the children of a dementia caregiver?

Let them talk, don't try to tell them what to do or how to handle something unless asked, offer to help if possible (particularly with transport), don't try to reason with them if they're upset about something or venting. Listen and be supportive.

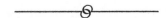

DREW:

Drew is our middle son. He was grown and living out of state during mom's illness. Drew is a trained minister and actually delivered marvelous funeral eulogies for both my parents. I'll be forever grateful to him for doing that. As one would expect from a minister, he is kind, understanding, and extremely insightful. Living out of state and working weekends in the church, his visits home to see mom were not as frequent as he would have liked. He would let me talk, and vent, to him for long periods of time via phone. Her changes were more pronounced for him than for those of us who saw her daily or weekly.

QUESTIONS & RESPONSES:

What was it like to watch Nana change during her dementia?

My perspective has to be different from everyone else in the family. They were all around Nana on a regular, if not daily basis, whereas I was living in a different state for the entirety of her diagnosis and battle with dementia. The decline was sharp to me, as I only saw and spoke with her once every few months. Seeing the change every time I came home was a challenge. She was a sharp and hard-working woman for as long as I had known her, so to see her struggle like that and become weaker and weaker was tough.

What do you think were the biggest impacts on me as her primary caregiver?

The impact that Nana's dementia had on you was significant. You were an only child, taking care of your mother who had been a rock for your entire life, while simultaneously working, being a mother of three, housing multiple foreign exchange students, and being a wife. All those titles, without adding caregiver to a parent with dementia are enough to challenge even the strongest person. Being Nana's primary caregiver just added to a significant amount of stress in your life. It wore you down and gave you less patience in the other areas and responsibilities in your life, which is no fault of your own. Anyone who has been in your shoes, or observed someone in your position, should understand the difficulty of being a primary caregiver. If I had to pick the two biggest impacts, they would be the emotional and mental toll that the caregiving took on you individually and the added stress to the marriage relationship.

How did this affect my relationship with you, short and long term?

Our relationship was not majorly impacted from my perspective. I could always sense the stress and pain that you were dealing with throughout the process. You often used our phone conversations as an outlet to vent and just get some thoughts out of your head. Listening is a skill set that just seems to be lost these days, and while

I know I should have talked to you more throughout the duration of Nana's battle with dementia, I tried to avoid rushing the conversations that we did have. On the short-term scale, it just revolves around the exhausted state that being a primary caregiver put you in. I never doubted your love for me and understood that your patience was going to be thin. As far as long term effects, I think that the strain and stress that you felt from the entire process has led you to stress about how the same scenario could happen between us if you or dad are diagnosed with dementia. I imagine it is part of the reason you were motivated to write this book.

How did this experience impact you personally, both positive and negative?

On the personal side of things, I'd say the experience challenged me to be present more with people, especially those who are older in my life. As a kid, I never really desired to have extended conversations with Nana or Papa (spelling?), but as I got older and less narcissistic, I realized how important and special those conversations were. I should have visited home more often than I did during that time. I missed out on some conversations with Nana and opportunities to support everyone else who was watching the dementia destroy Nana daily. There is that cliché phrase that people hold on just long enough to let those closest to them say goodbye. It had been months since I had been able to see Nana. She passed away less than 12 hours after I saw her for the last time. I'll never be able to forget seeing someone who had been so strong and independent in such a weak state. The experience overall just challenged me to invest more in the lives of those who are closest to me.

What is your best advice to the children of a dementia caregiver?

My best advice is simple. Remember that what your parent is going through is not easy. Many of the fights that you have will be a direct result of the exhaustion and stress that results from being a primary dementia caregiver. Always remember that you are not the center of the universe and until you have been the primary caregiver of someone you love who has dementia, you will not be able to understand that burden. Tell your parent(s) "I love you," cook dinner, ask to do things as a family, clean up the house, or offer to do whatever is asked to be of assistance.

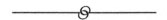

ETHAN:

Ethan is our youngest son and was in high school during my caregiving days. A three-sport athlete and singer, he was always quite busy and provided mom with much joy as she attended his various games and concerts. Frankly, while it made life more challenging to manage, his activities also provided a very welcome distraction for us. He was a teenager; his viewpoint now differs from his perspective then. I know he tried to interact with her well, but since she lived with us it was hard to watch her decline. He's now graduated college and is engaged to be married.

QUESTIONS & RESPONSES:

What was it like to watch Nana change during her dementia?

For this question, it's hard for me to answer because I just immersed myself into school, sports, and picking a college to really avoid doing anything. It was, I think I can say, interesting because of how up and down she would be, but I think it was also just heartbreaking to see. Part of the reason I avoided it is because there was a part of me that wanted her to be able to die to make it easier for you, and so she wouldn't be in pain; but either way, I knew there was going to be pain and those thoughts made me feel guilty.

What do you think were the biggest impacts on me as her primary caregiver?

I think the biggest impacts on you were it just made it harder for you to be who you are. And, more so, I think the bigger impacts came after Nana died. It felt like your identity had become wrapped up in taking care of her and especially because I was 18 and getting ready to go to college, you didn't really need to take care of me the way you did her. I could particularly tell on our vacation that summer, because you and dad were fighting constantly. So, I think the biggest impacts come after, not during.

How did this impact my relationship with you, short and long term?

Short term, I wanted to get away and since I was going to school that made it easier for me to do. It felt like walking on eggshells that summer [after her death] and it was frustrating; the memory of Nana and Papaw made it hard for me since I never dealt with my feelings. Long term, I saw how much you had sacrificed, and I know that I might be in the same position with you one day, so it made me have a greater appreciation for you and what you did.

How did this experience impact you personally, both positive and negative?

Honestly, I have yet to see anything positive, personally. That might be partly because I still haven't dealt with anything, but it just made me more confused about the world in general, and angry.

What is your best advice to the children of a dementia caregiver?

The best advice I could give is to just have a lot of patience and grace.

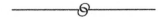

DAN:

Dan and I have been married since 1983. It's a special person who can be married to an only child like me, and he went above and beyond to serve me, our sons and my parents. At his initial invitation, my mom and dad sold their home and lived with us for over 12 years, until their deaths. An added challenge for him was that he has owned and operated his own professional service company from our home for most of our marriage. Dan was home every day with my parents, watching out for them, supporting me in my caregiving, and helping to bear the inherent burdens involved.

QUESTIONS & RESPONSES:

What was it like living with me (Toni) during my time as a dementia caregiver?

It was difficult, sad and frustrating. I was glad to help care for your mom. I tried to insure she took her meds, ate regularly, and didn't order a bunch of stuff from TV ads. I tried to sift through her repetitive comments for truth and her real needs and think of ways she could be helpful so she had a purpose. The situation was what it was, and there were things that needed to be done, so we did them.

What were the impacts you saw on me as a caregiver?

It took a big toll on you emotionally, physically and in time. There just weren't enough hours in the day. It wore you down, and you were tired and emotionally spent. It strengthened your bond with your mom, and you kept a pretty good attitude throughout the experience. There is so much coordination to do as a caregiver, and that has a big impact in many ways.

What was the impact on our marriage?

Short term, we didn't have much time together. I took over the logistics for Ethan [our youngest son who was 14 at the time] and handled more of the non-cooking and housework tasks. Long term, it ended up being the "cherry on top" of my already not being first in your life. This just pushed me further down the list. Because you had to devote so much of yourself to your mom's care, it built a greater emotional and physical distance between us. It hurt our relationship, and still does maybe for slightly different reasons.

What was the impact on you of my being mom's caregiver?

I became focused on helping you help her. Professionally, since I worked from home, it was a difficult time. My office was right above your dad's workshop in the basement, and 15 feet from their bedroom, which was where she spent almost all of her time. I always had one eye and ear on her - was she OK, was she doing something she shouldn't? It was tough with clients visiting, though it seemed to bother her much more than it did me. She was always afraid she was in the way. Regardless, she would interrupt my meetings or phone calls on occasion. Overall, it caused my servant nature to kick in, and I enjoyed helping her, and you, through that time.

What advice would you give the spouse/significant other of a caregiver?

Be supportive and patient. Make sure you plan time together away from your loved one, every 1-2 weeks. ASK for help from others and accept help when it is offered. Sitting with your loved one, bringing a meal, running errands are all very helpful and often are things the caregiver doesn't think of. They get so stuck on the caregiver track, it can be on autopilot. Understand that this is likely a short-term situation. There may be some long-term changes, but most things will return to normal. Make adjustments when needed and don't fret that it will be forever. If more changes are needed, make them. Know your boundaries, and pivot. Make sure the caregiver knows, without a doubt, that you are there to support them, not criticize, and that you love them...even when, especially when, they snap at you or others.

Notes

Chapters 1–5

[1] "Causes and Risk Factors for Alzheimer's Disease." Alzheimer's Association. https://www.alz.org/alzheimers-dementia/what-is-alzheimers/causes-and-risk-factors.

[2] Lanio, Charlene. "Mom Has Alzheimer's? Your Risk May Be High." WebMD. Last modified July 18, 2011. https://www.webmd.com/alzheimers/news/20110718/mom-has-alzheimers.

[3] "The Nine Enneagram Type Descriptions." The Enneagram Institute. https://www.enneagraminstitute.com/type-descriptions.

[4] "Dementia." Mayo Clinic. April 19, 2019. https://www.mayoclinic.org/diseases-conditions/dementia/symptoms-causes/syc-20352013.

[5] Karlawish, Jason, M.D. "Is It Dementia? Everyday Signs That Merit a Doctor Visit." AARP. Last modified June 25, 2018. https://www.aarp.org/health/dementia/info-2018/everyday-tasks-dementia-signs.html.

[6] "Types of Dementia." Alzheimer's Association. https://www.alz.org/alzheimers-dementia/what-is-dementia/types-of-dementia.

[7] "Dementia." Mayo Clinic. April 19, 2019. https://www.mayoclinic.org/diseases-conditions/dementia/symptoms-causes/syc-20352013.

[8] "Cognitive Assessment Toolkit." Alzheimer's Association.
https://www.alz.org/media/Documents/cognitive-assessment-toolkit.pdf.

[9] Lanphier, Loretta, NP, CN, CH, HHP. "11 Areas to Investigate before
Accepting a Dementia or Alzheimer's Diagnosis." Oasis Advanced
Wellness Health. Last modified June 27, 2017.
https://oawhealth.com/2017/06/27/11-areas-to-investigate-before-
accepting-a-dementia-or-alzheimers-diagnosis/.

[10] Gould, Elizabeth, MSW, LCSW, Stephanie Hughes, MPP, Michael
Lepore, PhD, and Joshua M. Wiener, PhD. "Research on Care
Coordination for People with Dementia and Family Caregivers." ASPE.
Last modified April 2017. https://aspe.hhs.gov/basic-report/research-care-
coordination-people-dementia-and-family-caregivers.

[11] Dictionary.com. https://www.dictionary.com/browse/cope?s=t.

[12] "Expectations Are Premeditated Resentments." Purple Treatment.
January 2017.
https://www.purpletreatment.com/journal/2017/1/2/expectations-are-
premeditated-resentments.

[13] Karlawish, Jason, M.D. "Is It Dementia? Everyday Signs That Merit a
Doctor Visit." AARP. Last modified June 25, 2018.
https://www.aarp.org/health/dementia/info-2018/everyday-tasks-
dementia-signs.html..

[14] Kan, Deborah. "Personality, Not Memory, Can Be Dementia's Greatest
Loss." Being Patient. Last modified September 2018.
https://www.beingpatient.com/personality-changes-dementia/.

[15] Graff-Radford, Jonathan, M.D. "Sundowning: Late-day Confusion."
Mayo Clinic. Last modified April 2019.
https://www.mayoclinic.org/diseases-conditions/alzheimers-disease/expert-
answers/sundowning/faq-20058511.

[16] "What does it mean to stepped out of a band box?" Answers. Last
modified November 2011.

https://www.answers.com/Q/What_does_it_mean_to_stepped_out_of_a_
band_box..

[17] "Still Alice." IMDB. https://www.imdb.com/title/tt3316960/.

Chapters 6–11

[18] "2020 Alzheimer's Disease Facts and Figures." Alzheimer's Association.
2020. https://www.alz.org/media/Documents/alzheimers-facts-and-
figures.pdf.

[19] "Stages of Alzheimer's & Dementia: Durations & Scales Used to
Measure Progression (GDS, FAST & CDR)." Dementia Care Central.
April 2020.
https://www.dementiacarecentral.com/aboutdementia/facts/stages/.

[20] "2020 Estate Planning and Wills Study." Caring.com. 2020.
https://www.caring.com/caregivers/estate-planning/wills-survey.

[21] Cummins, Eleanor. "Why Millennials are the 'Death Positive'
Generation." Vox. January 2020. https://www.vox.com/the-
highlight/2020/1/15/21059189/death-millennials-funeral-planning-
cremation-green-positive.

[22] Genworth. https://www.genworth.com/aging-and-you/finances/cost-of-
care.html.

[23] Shapiro, Joseph. "A New Nursing Home Population: The Young."
NPR. December 9, 2010.
https://www.npr.org/2010/12/09/131912529/a-new-nursing-home-
population-the-young.

[24] "Zoey's Extraordinary Playlist." NBC. https://www.nbc.com/zoeys-
extraordinary-playlist.

[25] Nicholas Sparks. https://nicholassparks.com/stories/the-notebook/.

26 "It's Time to Become Dementia Friendly." Alzheimer's Speaks. https://www.alzheimersspeaks.com/.

27 Bey, Lori La. "Your Memory Chip- Exercise." Alzheimer's Speaks. Last modified July 2009. https://alzheimersspeaks.wordpress.com/2009/07/27/your-memory-chip/.

28 Bey, Lori La. "Your Memory Chip- Exercise." Alzheimer's Speaks. Last modified July 2009. https://alzheimersspeaks.wordpress.com/2009/07/27/your-memory-chip/.

29 Joseph, Jenny. "Warning." Scottish Poetry Library. Last modified 1992. https://www.scottishpoetrylibrary.org.uk/poem/warning/..

30 "Still Alice." Rotten Tomatoes. https://www.rottentomatoes.com/m/still_alice.

31 "Sleep and Growing Older." Sleep Education. Last modified 2013. http://sleepeducation.org/news/2013/08/07/sleep-and-growing-older..

32 IMDb. https://www.imdb.com/title/tt1007029/.

33 "Positive Thinking: Stop Negative Self-talk to Reduce Stress." Mayo Clinic. https://www.mayoclinic.org/healthy-lifestyle/stress-management/in-depth/positive-thinking/art-20043950.

34 Netflix. https://www.netflix.com/title/70243583.

35 Ludden, David. "4 Reasons Why We Forget People's Names." Psychology Today. September 2017. https://www.psychologytoday.com/us/blog/talking-apes/201709/4-reasons-why-we-forget-peoples-names.

36 Shutterfly. https://www.shutterfly.com/.

37 "Ac-cent-tchu-ate the Positive." American Song Book. http://greatamericansongbook.net/pages/songs/a/accent-positive.html.

Chapters 12–18

[38] "Stress in America 2019." American Psychological Association. 2019. https://www.apa.org/news/press/releases/stress/2019/stress-america-2019.pdf.

[39] "Caregiver Stress." Alzheimer's Association. https://www.alz.org/help-support/caregiving/caregiver-health/caregiver-stress.

[40] Bannister, Craig. "Flashback-NFL Hall of Famer Gale Sayers: 'I Am Third,' Behind God and My Friends." CNS News. Last modified January 2018. https://www.cnsnews.com/blog/craig-bannister/flashback-nfl-hall-famer-gale-sayer-i-am-third-behind-god-and-my-friends.

[41] "Time spent working by full- and part-time status, gender, and location in 2014." U.S. Bureau of Labor Statistics. July 2015. https://www.bls.gov/opub/ted/2015/time-spent-working-by-full-and-part-time-status-gender-and-location-in-2014.htm.

[42] "Help for Caregivers." Caregiver Action Network. https://caregiveraction.org/resources/caregiver-statistics.

[43] Joy's House. https://joyshouse.org/.

[44] "Caregiving." Centers for Disease Control and Prevention. https://www.cdc.gov/aging/data/pdf/Aggregated-2017-caregiving-h.pdf.

[45] Jones, Derek. "Seniors Fear Nursing Home More than Death." Clear Care. June 2013. https://www.clearcareonline.com/blog/managing-a-homecare-agency/seniors-fear-nursing-home-more-than-death/.

[46] Howley, Elaine K. "Assisted Living Versus Senior Home Care." U.S. News. Last modified August 2019. https://health.usnews.com/best-assisted-living/articles/assisted-living-versus-senior-home-care.

[47] "Cost of Care Survey." Genworth. https://www.genworth.com/aging-and-you/finances/cost-of-care.html.

[48] "SNF Care past 100 Days." Medicare Interactive. https://www.medicareinteractive.org/get-answers/medicare-covered-services/skilled-nursing-facility-snf-services/snf-care-past-100-days#.

[49] "How to Apply for Medicaid and CHIP." USA Gov. https://www.usa.gov/medicaid.

[50] Snider, Natalie. "Home Matters: Aging in Place Housing Survey." AARP. March 2016. https://states.aarp.org/virginia/home-matters-survey.

[51] "Find a Nursing Home." U.S. News. https://health.usnews.com/best-nursing-homes.

[52] Day, Thomas. "About Nursing Homes." National Care Planning Council. https://www.longtermcarelink.net/eldercare/nursing_home.htm.

[53] Bernanzzani, Sophia. "Comparing End-of-Life Care Options." Aging Care. April 2020. https://www.agingcare.com/articles/comparing-end-of-life-care-options-198129.htm.

[54] "NHPCO Facts and Figures." National Hospice and Palliative Care Organization. 2018. https://www.nhpco.org/wp-content/uploads/2019/07/2018_NHPCO_Facts_Figures.pdf.

[55] Assisted Living Today. https://assistedlivingtoday.com/.

[56] Aging Care. https://www.agingcare.com/.

[57] Huntsberry- Lett, Ashley. End-of-Life Care: Signs That Death is Near. Aging Care. June 2020. https://www.agingcare.com/articles/end-of-life-care-signs-that-death-is-near-443741.htm.

[58] Silverstein, Shel. "Snowball." All Poetry. https://allpoetry.com/poem/8538951-Snowball-by-Shel-Silverstein.

[59] Brown, Malika. "Dealing with Caregiver Guilt." Caregiver. https://caregiver.com/articles/dealing-caregiver-guilt/.

60 Kuffel, Hunter, CEFP. "How Long Does An Executor Have To Distribute a Will?" SmartAsset. March 13, 2019. https://smartasset.com/estate-planning/how-long-does-executor-have-to-distribute-will.

61 Caring Bridge. https://www.caringbridge.org/.

62 "19 Inspirational Quotes About Hope and Healing." Caring Bridge. March 2018. https://www.caringbridge.org/resources/inspirational-quotes-about-hope-healing/.

63 Ott, Carol H., Sara Sanders, and Sheryl T. Kelber. "Grief and Personal Growth Experience of Spouses and Adult-Child Caregivers of Individuals with Alzheimer's Disease and Related Dementias." The Gerontologist 47, no. 6 (December 2007): 798–809. https://doi.org/10.1093/geront/47.6.798.

64 Feldman, David B. "Why the Five Stages of Grief Are Wrong." Psychology Today. Last modified July 2017. https://www.psychologytoday.com/us/blog/supersurvivors/201707/why-the-five-stages-grief-are-wrong.

65 "Grief and Loss." Family Caregiver Alliance. https://www.caregiver.org/grief-and-loss.

66 Nicholas Sparks. https://nicholassparks.com/stories/the-notebook/.

67 "Harry Potter and the Chamber of Secrets: Summary." Spark Notes. https://www.sparknotes.com/lit/potter2/summary/.

68 "How Crying can make you Healthier." Independent. https://www.independent.co.uk/life-style/health-and-families/features/how-crying-can-make-you-healthier-1009169.html.

69 Go Ahead, Have a Good Cry: 5 Reasons Why It's Good for You." Aging Care. October 2019. https://www.agingcare.com/articles/reasons-why-crying-is-good-for-your-health-146022.htm.

[70] "How Crying Can Make You Healthier." Independent.
https://www.independent.co.uk/life-style/health-and-
families/features/how-crying-can-make-you-healthier-1009169.html.

[71] Govender, Serusha. "Crying: The Health Benefits of Tears." Web MD.
https://www.webmd.com/balance/features/is-crying-good-for-you#1.

[72] "Harry Potter and the Half Blood Prince: Plot Overview." Spark Notes.
https://www.sparknotes.com/lit/potter6/summary/.

[73] "12 Steps in Grief Process." Dennis Toll Funeral Home.
https://dennistoll.ca/12_Steps_in_Grief_Process_981014.html.

Resources*

Apps for Dementia Patient Engagement

- AmuseIT – prompts memories and conversation, helps engagement
- Flower Garden - grow flowers and send bouquets
- It's Done – remember later what you do now
- Jigsaw Puzzles Real – adjust pieces from 9 to 1000
- Let's Create! Pottery – throw clay and make virtual clay pots
- Luminosity: Brain Training – science based to exercise brain
- MindMate - memory tests, workouts & food
- MyReef 3D Aquarium – interact with fish
- Piano with Songs – play piano virtually
- Spaced Retrieval Therapy - helps recall important information

Caregiver Support

- AARP (www.aarp.org)
- Alzheimer's Association (www.alz.org)
- Alzheimer's Foundation of America (www.seniorlink.com)
- Alzheimers.net (www.alzheimers.net)
- Alzheimer's Speaks (www.alzheimersspeaks.com)
- ARCH National Respite Network (www.archrespite.org)
- Bambu Care (www.letsbambu.com)
- Being Patient (www.beingpatient.com)
- Caregiver Action Network (www.caregiveraction.org)
- CareLinx (www.kindlycare.com)
- Caring.com (www.caring.com)
- CaringBridge (www.caringbridge.org)
- Clear Care (www.clearcareonline.com)
- Cleveland Clinic/Healthy Brains (www.healthybrains.org)
- Daily Caring (www.dailycaring.com)
- Dementia Friendly America (www.dfamerica.org)
- Dementia Society of America (www.memorycafedirectory.com)
- Family Caregiver Alliance (www.caregiver.org)
- Live Better With (www.livebetterwith.com)
- Mended Hearts (www.mended-hearts.org)
- National Alliance for Caregiving (www.caregiving.org)
- National Association of Area Agencies on Aging (www.n4a.org)
- National Institute on Aging (www.nia.nih.gov)
- Psychology Today (www.psychologytoday.com)
- U.S. Department of Veterans Affairs (www.va.gov)

Dementia, Diseases & Aging

- Alzheimers.net (www.alzheimers.net)
- American Academy of Hospice and Palliative Medicine (www.palliativedoctors.org)
- American Cancer Society (www.cancer.org)
- American Diabetes Association (www.diabetes.org)
- American Heart Association (www.heart.org)
- American Stroke Association (www.strokeassociation.org)
- Centers for Disease Control and Prevention (www.cdc.gov)
- The Gerontological Society of America (https://www.geron.org)
- Mayo Clinic (www.mayoclinic.org)
- National Parkinson's Foundation (www.parkinson.org)
- Oasis Advanced Wellness (www.oawhealth.com)
- The Michael J. Fox Foundation for Parkinson's Research (www.michaeljfox.org)
- U.S. Department of Health and Human Services (www.aspe.hhs.gov)
- WebMD (www.webmd.com)

Financial & Legal

- Alzheimer's Foundation of America (www.seniorlink.com)
- American Association for Long-Term Care Insurance (www.aaltci.org)
- Center for Medicare Advocacy (www.medicareadvocacy.org)

- Dementia Care Central
  (https://www.dementiacarecentral.com/financial-planning/alzheimers/)
- ElderLaw Answers (www.elderlawanswers.com)
- Forbes (www.forbes.com)
- Genworth (www.genworth.com)
- Kiplinger (https://www.kiplinger.com/financial-planning-for-alzheimers)
- Medicaid (www.medicaid.gov)
- Medicare (www.medicare.gov)
- Medicare Interactive (www.medicareinteractive.org)
- National Institute on Aging (www.nia.nih.gov)
- SeniorAdvisor.com (www.senioradvisor.com)

Patient Care & Residential Options

- a Place for Mom (www.aplaceformom.com)
- Abe's Garden (www.abesgarden.org)
- American Health Care Association (www.ahcancal.org)
- AssistedLiving.org (www.assistedlivingtoday.com)
- CareLinx/KindlyCare (www.dailycaring.com)
- Centers for Medicare & Medicaid Services
  (www.medicare.gov)
- Hospice Foundation of America
  (www.hospicefoundation.org)
- Joy's House (www.joyshouse.org)
- National Adult Day Services Association (www.nadsa.org)
- National Hospice and Palliative Care Organization
  (www.nhpco.org)
- Visiting Angels (www.visitingangels.com)
- Senior Advisor (www.locate.senioradvisor.com)

Patient Support & Activities

- 6-Minute Fitness (www.sixminutefitness.com) exercises for fitness at 60+
- Alz Calls (www.alzcalls.com) record your voice, add a photo and a chatbot responds to your loved one with live interactive conversation when you are not able to respond to repeated calls
- AngelSense GPS (www.angelsense.com/gps-tracker-for-elderly)
- Benjamin Rose Institute on Aging (https://benrose.org/)
- Caregiver Matters (www.medicareadvocacy.org)
- Daily Caring (www.dailycaring.com)
- Keeping Busy www.keepingbusy.com) site with activities for patients
- MedicAlert + Safe Return (www.alz.org/help-support/caregiving/safety/medicalert-with-24-7-wandering-support)
- Medical Guardian (www.medicalguardian.com) alert system
- Memory Health (www.dailycaring.com)
- MEternally (www.meternally.com) photo and activity cards, tools to promote memory
- Mobile Help (www.mobilehelp.com) alert system
- National Care Planning Council (www.longtermcarelink.net)
- The Conversation Project (www.theconversationproject.org)

Podcasts about dementia and caregiving

- Podcast: Happy Healthy Caregiver
  (www.thewholecarenetwork.com/happyhealthycaregiver)
- Podcast: Life With Dementia
  (https://lifewithdementia.libsyn.com/)
- Podcast: This Dementia Life
  (https://lifewithdementia.libsyn.com/)
- Podcast: What The Dementia
  (https://anchor.fm/whatthedementia)

Recommended Further Reading

- *The Splendor of Babies: A Picture Book for Seniors, Adults with Alzheimer's and Others,* Emma Rose Sparrow; Sterling Elle Publishing, 2015. (Picture book for patients).
- *The 36-Hour Day: A Family's Guide to Caring for People Who Have Alzheimer's Disease, Related Dementias, and Memory Loss,* 6th edition, Nancy L. Mace and Peter V. Rabins; Johns Hopkins University Press, 2017.
- *Chicken Soup for the Caregiver's Soul: Stories to Inspire Caregivers in the Home, Community and the World,* Jack Canfield, Mark Victor Hansen, LeAnn Thieman; Chicken Soup for the Soul Publishing, 2012.
- *Creating Moments of Joy Along the Alzheimer's Journey: A Guide for Families and Caregivers,* 5th edition, Jolene Brackey; Purdue University Press, 2016.
- *Before I Forget,* B. Smith, Dan Gasby; Harmony Books, 2016.
- *Finding Grace in the Face of Dementia,* John Dunlop, M.D.; Crossway, 2017.
- *Passages in Caregiving: Turning Chaos into Confidence,* Gail Sheehy; Harper, 2011.
- *The Alzheimer's Solution: A Breakthrough Program to Prevent and Reverse the Symptoms of Cognitive Decline at Every Age,* Dean Sherzai M.D., Ayesha Sherzai M.D.; Harper One, 2019.

- *When Reasoning No Longer Works: A Practical Guide for Caregivers Dealing with Dementia & Alzheimer's Care,* 2nd edition, Angel Smits; Parker Hayden Media, 2017.
- *Grandma and Me: A Kid's Guide for Alzheimer's and Dementia,* Beatrice Tauber Prior Psy.D., Mary Ann Drummond RN, et, al.; Morgan James Publishing, 2018.
- *Connecting Memories – Book 1: A Coloring Book for Adults with Dementia-Alzheimer's (Volume 1),* 2nd edition, Bonnie S. MacLachlan; Art Z. Illustrations, 2016.

Acknowledgements

I've heard that nearly 90% of people want to write a book. Only 3% of them actually do. Being an author sounds so glamorous. When I was in elementary school, I wrote a story about a snowman and Santa. My teacher whispered in my ear that she was sure one day I'd write a book. I can't say I gave that prediction much thought since. In looking back over my life, I have written a lot, about a variety of topics. Vignettes, devotions and newsletter articles for my church. Blogs and webpages for my jobs. Essays for…well, I wasn't sure what for. But I was compelled to record my thoughts in case they would be useful someday. Always be prepared, you know.

Now, I find myself an author. Publishing a book is a tremendous accomplishment that doesn't happen without lots of encouragement and support. I am compelled once again to record my thoughts, and my gratitude, for those who have helped me through this journey.

First, I thank my saint of a husband, Dan, who invited my parents to live with our family and then patiently survived twelve years of their quirks, squabbles and eventual disease. He took a backseat as I became my mom's caregiver and didn't complain once. He supported me, encouraged, served as de facto editor, title guru and idea man, ordered dinner out more times than I can count – anything that would help me have margin to write. Dan tells it like it is, which is both painful and freeing. I could not have completed this without his love and encouragement. I can never tell him thank you, and I love you, enough.

My three sons, Adam, Drew and Ethan, daughter-in-law Hayleigh and daughter-in-law to be Cassidy have been great cheerleaders. Each in their own way has provided direction, ideas, editing and inspiration. The original purpose for recording my caregiving experiences was to help them confidently know how to care for me if needed, with much less stress and difficulty. Without that foundational "mother bear" focus, I may never have had the strength to author this book.

Several professionals have been involved with this effort. Self Publishing School (SPS), Chandler Bolt, Sean Sumner and Scott Allan have coached me from idea to publication. They taught me to celebrate everything, not give up, and believe in my abilities in this new career. My fellow writers in the SPS Mastermind answered questions, gave advice, and cheered me on. My production team – Sky Nuttall (editing), Angie Ayala at pro_ebookscovers (cover design), and Jason & Marina Anderson at Polgarus Studio (formatting) – put the polishing touches on an otherwise rookie endeavor. I am so grateful for their expertise, professionalism and support.

Finally, and most importantly, I must thank Jesus Christ. It is through Him alone that I had the strength to wear the caregiver mantle. He protected me and Nana from the devastating discouragement that is often part of this disease. I am humbled by that reality. My best, and only, response is to share what I learned with others, to encourage them as I was encouraged. I want you to see beyond your challenges on this journey to the LIFE that is available every day.

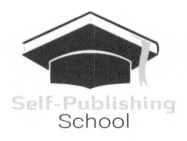

Self-Publishing
School

NOW IT'S YOUR TURN

**Discover the EXACT 3-step blueprint you need to become
a bestselling author in as little as 3 months.**

Self-Publishing School helped me, and now I want them to help
you with this FREE resource to begin outlining your book!

Even if you're busy, bad at writing, or don't know where to start,
you CAN write a bestseller and build your best life.

With tools and experience across a variety of niches and professions,
Self-Publishing School is the <u>only</u> resource you need to
take your book to the finish line!

DON'T WAIT

Say "YES" to becoming a bestseller:

https://self-publishingschool.com/friend/

Follow the steps on the page to get a FREE resource to get started
on your book and unlock a discount to get started with Self-
Publishing School

About the Author

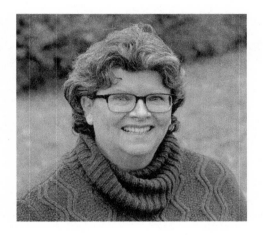

Toni Kanzler wears several hats: wife, mother, CPA, entrepreneur, private school administrator, non-profit volunteer and board member. But it was her daughter hat that brought the privilege of being her mother's caregiver. Toni is passionate about helping others have greater confidence, less stress, and to experience joy in their caregiving journey.

Watch for Toni's future publications meant to encourage you to look beyond the obvious to see the truth that lives in the ordinary...and extraordinary.

Can You Help?

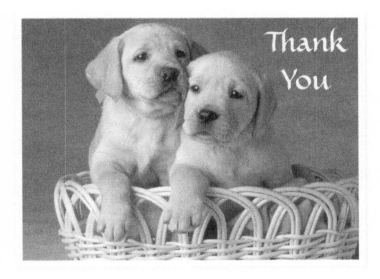

Thank You for Reading My Book!

I would love to have your feedback.

Your input will help me make the next version of this book and my future books the best they can be.

Please leave me an honest review on Amazon letting me know what you thought of the book - did it accomplish my goal of encouraging and equipping you as a caregiver.

Thanks so much!

Toni Kanzler

Made in the USA
Las Vegas, NV
01 October 2021